Gender and Health

# Gender and Health

Madhu Nagla

RAWAT PUBLICATIONS
Jaipur • New Delhi • Bangalore • Guwahati • Kolkata

ISBN 978-81-316-0578-3



**Reprinted, 2016**



*Publishedby*
Prem Rawat for **Rawat Publications**
Satyam Apts, Sector 3, Jawahar Nagar, Jaipur 302 004 (India)
Phone: 0141 265 1748 / 7006 Fax: 0141 265 1748
E-mail: info@rawatbooks.com
Website: www.rawatbooks.com

*New Delhi Office*
4858/24, Ansari Road, Daryaganj, New Delhi 110 002
Phone: 011 2326 3290

Also at *Bangalore, Guwahati* and *Kolkata*

Typeset by Rawat Computers, Jaipur
Printed and bound in India

Dedicated to my grandson
ABHIGYAN

# Contents

# Preface

This book *Gender and Health* is a collection of 11 articles which were published in various national and international journals and edited books over a period of time. The book examines, within the broad context of women's health, issues pertaining their health and rights, medical encounters, and different laws designed to meet their health needs, specifically reproductive and mental health.

The health of a country's women population has deep implications for the health and development of children, their future well-being and also for women themselves. Poor health, undernutrition among females results in high mortality, morbidity, and stunt growth of children and women during their life cycle.

The gender inequality entrenched in our social structure manifested through patriarchal structure puts women in an unequal position in terms of health indicators. This health inequality is depicted in the reproductive behaviour, and several encounters while seeking health. The effects of pervasive health are also explained in various laws, rights and ethics, which are directly concerned to women. The health of girl child and her survival, in fact, depends on the woman's health and her nutritional status.

Feeling of suffering is influenced/conditioned by the female's self-denial/neglect psychology, governed by the patriarchal norms, especially when the suffering is mild. High priority to household work and low priority to health also affect a woman's health-seeking behaviour. They need permission and escort to visit health centre. Institution-based health system generates inhibitions among the illiterate rural women about the alien environment of the hospital, and the patriarchal bias among the health providers increases such inhibition.

I take this opportunity to thank my academic friends who had enriched me with their knowledge base on various health issues. Frequent interactions with my teachers and colleagues from all corners helped me immensely ever since I thought of writing this book. I also take this opportunity to thank Rawat Publications for constantly encouraging me to write on this subject and accepting manuscript for publication.

I would also like to thank my family which includes, my son Gaurav and daughter-in-law Archana, my daughter Radhika and son-in-law Rohit. Our lovely grandson, Abhigyan's birth was of enduring impressions and beautiful moments during my writing phase of book. Another important milestone in one's life takes place when you fulfil the dreams of your life partner. Bhupendra Kumar, my husband made all this possible with his love, understanding and support, by helping me overcome the troubling periods and for being patient throughout these years. Finally, its the Almighty's help that made all this work possible.

# Introduction

The concept of women's health covers mortality, morbidity, nutritional status and reproductive health. The health of a woman is conditioned by her social, cultural and economic status in the society. Women's experiences as recipients of health care and, to a lesser extent, their work as providers of health care have attracted a great deal of attention in the contemporary society. Although there are a number of fields directly concerned with the women and their health and started receiving attention in the gender debate.

Feminists today question both the level of women's health status and the quality of health care they receive, linking these problems to the extreme sexual segregation of the health care labour force, (e.g., male doctors and female nurses) as well as to some of the broader questions of political economy which they see as having influenced by these developments. Very early in the new era of feminists organizing health care, critics and their supporters argued that these matters were proper foci both for political action and for scholarly inquiry. Early works of these scholars include the classic *Our Bodies Our Selves* (Boston Women's Health Book Collective, 1973) and the writings of Seaman (1969, 1972), Ehrenreich and English (1972, 1973), Chesler (1972) and Frankfort (1972).

The focus of the book is to present a combination of theoretic frameworks and empirical realities. The various health issues discussed in the book include a growing inequality of health for women and girl child, women's health ethics and right issues, the impact of technology on the practice of delivery of health care, particularly obstetrical care, and the experiences of pregnant women. The state and laws governing the health of women are far more important as the future distribution of shrinking health resources also adversely affect the women. Demographic predictions point to the 'missing girl children' which is an important segment of the population. At the same time, observers of epidemiological and service-utilization trends have shown that women seem to experience illness more often than do men. The importance of these themes to the future direction of health care delivery as well as to the quality of life of the female population mandates a fresh approach to the analysis of women's health issues, and thus places them in a broad societal context.

In order to study the various aspects of health related to women, we need to study the various levels of health care, stages in a woman's life and also the providers of health care. Various interventions at the level of health policy are also dealt with. For a long time we have been studying the inequality of gender in general and also at specific level in terms of education, employment, wages, and of course health. However, in this book, we have tried to systematize the different stages in the life of a woman and her health concerns. These life stages start from girl child and move towards motherhood. The health concerns of a woman are related with her reproductive health, obstetrical care, health rights, mental health, nutritional intake and leisure-health activities. The inaccessibility of health care is also summarized in the form of state policy or at the level of lack of infrastructure. Many times, the apathy of doctors towards women also becomes the cause of deprivation of health care resources, which is also investigated.

The compilation of different themes related to women becomes further important as they are based on either empirical research work or on secondary sources of information. Some studies also offer certain narratives which enrich the qualitative base of the book.

The book begins with the paper on '*Gender, Health and Healing: Different Perspectives*' which presents theoretical approaches for studying health and gender. Different theoretical frameworks presented in the chapter for studying health and healing among women provide a base for understanding the health issues and relate it to the gender. The purpose is to provide a broader understanding of the phenomenon. Various alternative perspectives or overlapping perspectives provide enough scope to interpret the data generated from the study in generalized perspective. Schutz (1970: 5 cited by Sampson, 1976: 87) has rightly pointed out that 'all our knowledge of the world, in common sense as well as in scientific thinking, involves constructs, i.e., a set of abstractions, generalizations, formalizations, idealizations specific to the respective level of thought organisation … . Strictly speaking, here are no such things as facts, pure and simple. All facts are from the outset facts selected from a universal context by the activities of our mind. They are, therefore, always interpreted facts … .'

The second chapter on '*Gender Inequality: Perceptive Threat to Health*' in all its critical matters such as demographic features, access to health care delivery, nutritional pattern and family planning, is based on secondary data. It argues that the gender inequality exists in the meaning attached to illness, the interpretation of etiology and the action to be taken in dealing with illness of all kind.

In the next four chapters, we return to our overall theme that women's health should be considered in relation to other aspects of the society under discussion – and are thus able to determine state's response to the women's health issues. These include '*Gender Analysis and Population Issues*', '*Understanding Women's Health and Right Issues*', '*Women and Health Issues Under Law*', and '*Women and Ethics in Medicine: Historical Perspective and Contemporary Concern*'. Controversies over population policies concerning with the reproductive health in India have evoked discourse that how state and women may coerce differently of their fundamental interests. The health rights and laws for women reflect on broad characteristics and changes within the societies. As you can see, a number of issues are indicative of features of laws, rights and ethics and respond to the implications on women. The reciprocal influence of laws, rights and ethics reflects the actual construction of gender and health in society, as well as the nature of the society itself that we wish to stress, since we see these links as integral for the sound analysis of policy relevant for women's health.

The next four chapters, viz., '*Girl Child Health in India*', '*Obstetrical Care Decisions Among Village Women in Haryana*', '*Medical Encounters: The Experience of Illness and Treatment*', and '*Women and Mental Health: Disposition, Narratives and Treatment*' analyse the health care providers and receivers interaction pattern. Description in these chapters shows that how variously women's health and illness can be constructed and responded accordingly.

The last chapter on *'Yoga, Health and Leisure: Attitudes of Women in Haryana'* suggests that the domain of yoga leisure is denied to women, although, it contributes to the good health of women. It concludes that leisure, yoga and health among women are all embedded in the surrounding social contexts and, indeed, that leisure activities in general are inextricably entwined with their broader cultural and structural contexts.

This volume thus presents analysis of the above various themes not only in their own right, but, further, as they reflect on broad characteristics and changes within the Indian society across social variables. Number of health issues from the gender perspective are important and all the chapters tell us something about the specific problem at issue and about the wider society within which that problem is situated. It is the overall themes of reciprocal influence, between women's issues considered in their own right and what they reflect about the actual construction of gender and health in society, as well as the nature of the society itself that we wish to stress, since we see these links an integral for the sound analysis of policy relevant for women's health.

There are, of course, many other themes which we wish to include, however, by virtue of our limitation of a single volume we could not do the same. We would hope that such additions will be taken up in near future.

## References

Boston Women's Health Book Collective (1973), *Our Bodies Our Selves*, New York: Simon and Schuster.

Chesler, P. (1972), *Women and Madness*, Garden City, New York: Doubleday.

Ehrenreich, B. and D. English (1972), *Witches, Midwives and Nurses: A History of Women Healers*, Old Westbury, New York: Feminist Press.

——. (1973), *Complaints and Disorders: The Sexual Politics of Sickness*, Old Westbury, New York: Feminist Press.

Frankfort, E. (1972), *Vaginal Politics*, New York: Quadrangle Books.

Sampson, E.E. (1976), *Social Psychology and Comparative Society*, New York: John Wiley and Sons, Inc.

Seaman, B. (1969), *The Doctor's Case against the Pill*, New York: Avon.

——. (1972), *Free and Female*, New York: Coward, McCann and Geoghegan.

# 1 Gender, Health and Healing

## Different Perspectives

Sociological study often involves itself in investigating what appears at first sight to be natural, universal or common sense, only to discover that such behaviours or practices are fundamentally affected by specific social factors and influences. At the outset, any social phenomenon which appears to be natural or general or simply common however, when these phenomena or behaviours or incidents are put for sociological inquiry, they are affected by certain social factors or certain other causative actors.

The health and health services are not recent phenomena, they have their history. There is a plurality of systems of medicine in every society. However, in the contemporary society, the modern or scientific system of medicine is dominating. This modern system of medicine has also developed certain critiques or has been questioned by some users of the system. They argue that it has done more harm in comparison to its benefits. It can only be sorted out when we systematically proceed for its analysis by putting different approaches. For example, functional and conflict approaches acknowledge that health professionals, particularly doctors, possess a significant amount of power. They have great influence on the users. They not only treat the patients, but also have power to sanction sick leave, eligibility for different reimbursements of medicine and diagnostic expenditures. They also endorse controlling and restraining actions such as the incarceration of individuals defined as mentally ill.

While health services seem self-evidently beneficial, some have questioned their impact, even arguing that the harm done by modern medicine outweighs the benefits. We can explore the debate by distinguishing between consensus and conflict approaches. The functional approach suggests that health professionals' power is necessary for the smooth functioning of modern societies and establishes the coordination between the different elements of social structure. Health professionals are supposed to have an extensive and specialized professional training which subscribes the healing power among them. They have a commitment to ethical conduct and altruistic orientation which not only puts them in higher hierarchy of professionals but also allows them to carry out their service orientation. Opposed to it is the conflict perspective which questions the power of the health professionals and their domination over the patients. The dominance is exhibited in the form of social control and monopoly of subscription and diagnosis. This is also reflected in the form of unequal relationship between health professionals and patients.

Consensus approaches accept the necessity of these functions for the smooth running of modern societies. Furthermore, they suggest that members of regulated professions are, because of their extensive training and commitment to ethical conduct, well placed to carry them out. In contrast, conflict perspectives question professional power, highlighting issues of professional domination and social control, and the oppressive impact of some practices. Below we will be dealing with these approaches in detail.

## Functionalist Perspective

Talcott Parsons is regarded as one of the key proponents of the functional approach. In his writings (1951, 1975), he demonstrated the ways in which practices such as medicine contribute to the maintenance of the social order. He argues that illness not only disturbs individual functioning, but is also socially dysfunctional, undermining the values, activities and roles that support productivity and social stability. In order to prevent such a disruption, mechanisms are needed that render illness an undesirable and temporary social state. Parsons identified such a mechanisms in the form of sick role, into which people ideally enter when they become ill. Parsons depicted sick role as involving both rights and obligations.

The two rights are:

- An exemption from responsibilities such as work and social obligations, which needs to be legitimized by a physician in order to be valid.
- That the sick individuals avoid any blame or responsibility for their condition.

The two obligations are:

- The sick person must want to get better.
- The sick person must seek competent help, usually from a trained physician.

Now, the question arises: How adequate is the sick role in accounting for someone:

1. with food poisoning,
2. with depression,
3. with asthma,
4. who is HIV positive?

Parsons' sick role concept has stimulated an important debate on the role of medicine and the nature of medical power. Sociologists have debated the relevance of the concept in relation to contemporary patterns of health and illness.

One of the issues that arise is that access to the sick role may not be enjoyed equally by all. The sick role concept may apply relatively closely to acute illnesses such as influenza, but even in these cases there are some social obligations (such as caring for others) from which exemptions may be difficult to gain. In the case of chronic conditions, however, the rights associated with the sick role concept apply less clearly, and social obligations may be difficult to escape in the longer term. Furthermore, some conditions (for example, HIV/AIDS) carry a stigma. This means that assumptions of responsibility and blame may influence how the person is seen and treated by others.

The obligations associated with the sick role concept are also more complex than they appear. Sociologists have pointed out that these obligations render the doctor much more powerful than the patient in professional-client interactions. Functionalists such as Parsons accept the asymmetrical nature of the doctor-patient relationship on the ground that doctors, as modern professionals, are required to be altruistic. They are also expected to be committed to other professional values such as universalism, collectivism and neutrality. These values are seen as ensuring that a doctor's personal feelings towards a patient do not influence the consultation or treatment offered. The physician is expected to put the welfare of the patient above any personal interest.

The power misbalance between doctors and patient seems, however, less easy to accept if the professional commitment to these values is questioned. A more critical perspective would suggest that society, rather than being made of groups that share equal access to power, is made up of groups with competing interests and unequal influence and these include professionals, whose interests may conflict with those of patients. From this perspective, the degree of autonomy and the lack of external surveillance of many procedures is questionable. This position of professional autonomy, it is argued, protects the doctor from scrutiny and expresses the patient to potential abuse.

Although the sick role concept has been widely criticized, however, it has provided a useful insight into the experience of illness and the role of medicine. Importantly, it has drawn attention to questions of power, paving the way for a broader debate on the nature of medical authority and the relationship between medicine and social control.

## Medicalization and Social Control

During the 1960 and 70s, a number of critical perspectives on medical power emerged. These often drew on the medicalization thesis, in which medicine is seen as expanding its social jurisdiction and replacing earlier mechanisms of social control such as religion. While Parsons' functionalist model emphasized the benign and productive aspects of medical power, critical perspectives have identified some undesirable social costs of medical expansion.

The medicalization of society has been seen as taking place at a number of levels (Zola, 1972):

- Medicine has expanded its concerns to encompass areas of life not previously regarded as illness.
- Medicalization has resulted in the concentration of control over technical procedures among doctors.
- Doctors' authority has expanded to encompass areas of moral decision-making.

Medicalization involves the pursuit of medical, individual and technical solutions to an expanding range of problems. Where these problems are social in origin, medicalization can be seen as obscuring their social causes, inhibiting the development of alternative solutions.

## Medicine as a Threat to Health

In one well-known critique, Illich (1977) described medicalization as a major threat to health. Modern medicine was portrayed as generating iatrogenic disease that is illness that would have not come about without medical intervention. It was also suggested that society would be better off without professions such as medicine, which encourage dependency rather than self-reliance.

While it seems unethical to suggest that people be denied access to medical treatment, Illich's ideas remain influential. Contemporary journalism often seeks to expose the 'dangers of modern medicine', while the increasing popularity of complementary therapies and widespread disillusionment with conventional medical approaches.

Illich's ideas also continue to be debated in academic circles. One critique revisits the concept of iatrogenesis in relation to the negative impact of conventional health care on women. Foster (1995) suggests that the benefits of modern medicine are oversold and its harmful effects understated. As patients, women are constrained in their ability to make rational choices, partly because doctors are themselves unaware of many of the risks attached to accepted forms of medical treatment. Furthermore, when doctors are aware of the risks, they may assume that female patients will not be able to cope with the information, and therefore keep their knowledge to themselves (Foster, 1995; Illich, 1975, 1977; McTaggart, 1996).

It is important not to overstate the benefits of medical practice, but these theories may understate medicine's benefits; empirical evidence is needed in order to evaluate the impact of different health interventions. Furthermore, these theories imply that attempts to reduce inequalities in health by widening the access to medical intervention are not worthwhile since these will simply extended rather than address the problem. Given that, for many people in the world, access to basic health care is limited, it seems important to emphasize widening access to beneficial practices and resources as well as re-examine questionable aspects of medical practice.

These theories do, however, highlight the impact of medical decision-making and point towards the need for a greater involvement of patients and lay people in such activity. In the face of such challenging claims about medicine, it seems that consumers need to make more and more complex and difficult choices concerning their health care.

Now, we move on to the approaches to understand relationship between medicine, health professions and society.

## Marxist and Political Economy Perspectives

These perspectives also highlight the negative impact of medical power. However, rather than seeing professions as the main problem, Marxist theory suggests that professional power is a product of a deeper set of power relations. Political economy perspective, also drawn on Marxist theory, suggests that the structure of society around the needs of capitalism as an economic system is the starting point of any analysis of health and health care. This theory suggests that capitalist societies are organized around the generation of profit, which is created by exploitation of labour power.

Political economy writers such as Doyal (1979) and Navarro (1979) drew broadly on this theory and applied to health in a number of ways as under:

- The processes of industrial capitalism cause ill health directly, for example, through occupational disease, industrial accidents and the manufacturing and marketing of harmful consumer products.
- The burden of disease is disproportionately felt by those in lower socio-economic groups.
- Society does not do enough to prevent these problems or promote health because its resources are channelled towards the maintenance of production over and above the social goal of securing and improving public health.

According to Navarro (1979), doctors are, partly because of their own class position and partly because of their social role, often seen as serving the interests of the dominant class. Hence, the role of medicine is seen as helping to minimize disruption to the economic functioning of society, even if this means supporting exploitative and oppressive economic and social relationships.

Now, a question arises: How relevant is the view that capitalism is a major threat to population health?

The global nature of capitalism makes it perhaps impossible to identify examples of societies and cultures unaffected by it. However, critics have argued that social processes, other than the economic ones, emphasized by Marxist writers, are equally influential. These include the movement of ideas and discourses. Furthermore, critics have also argued that Marxism places too much emphasis on class divisions as the driving forces of social change, ignoring the independent impact of other social relations, including gender and ethnicity.

In response to these criticisms, political economy perspective has taken a broader view than those of traditional Marxism, widening their scope to examine other aspects of power relationships such as gender and ethnicity. Political economy perspective has exercised a strong influence over the sociology of health and illness, although this influenced declined during the 1980s and 90s as new economic and social trends, such as changes in employment, leisure and lifestyle, emerged to challenge core assumptions concerning identity and class. Political economy perspective may still evolve to meet these challenges. In the meantime, however, their legacy can still be seen, for example, in relation to the inequalities in health debate, where material and structural explanations continue to hold sway.

## Interactionist Perspective and the Experience of Illness

The perspectives discussed so far concentrate on the impact of illness, health and health care on society as a whole. Sociologists have also examined the nature and meaning of the illness experience at the individual level, analysing it in the context of the interaction between people and exploring its implication for notions of identity and self. This tradition draws on the work of George Herbert Mead (1934), who saw human beings as distinctive in that they are able to reflect on their own thoughts and actions. This approach, sometimes referred to as 'symbolic interactionism', emphasizes the ways in which people gain a shared understanding of the meanings, attached to objects and phenomena, which are not seen as pre-existing or intrinsic. Instead, they emerge from an interpretative process between people in which language is an important element. A nurse's uniform, for example, suggests feminity, caring, altruism and sacrifice – meanings reaffirmed by countless media portrayals.

Sociologists have applied these insights to the study of changes in identity, which occur when people become chronically ill or impaired. Goffman's work on Stigma (1963) provides a well-known example of such an approach. According to him, a person's sense of identity is formed in interaction with others and is strongly influenced by other people's perceptions. These are reflected back to the individual through verbal and non-verbal communication. When someone possesses a distinguishing attribute that is perceived negatively by others, his or her identity is to some extent 'spoiled' by the stigma. People attribute a range of negative characteristics, not necessarily directly related to the original attribute, to the individual. Wheelchair users, for example, are often assumed to be physically and intellectually dependent. Stigma is not just attributed to people on the basis of physical attributes, but can also be attributed as a result of personal and social characteristics such as being gay or lesbian.

Goffman suggested that, once stigmatized, individuals may react in a number of ways. They may attempt to 'pass', maintaining a performance of self in which the stigmatized attribute is disguised or hidden. They may also respond in ways that seem to confirm society's stereotyped views. Alternatively, they may create meanings that turn their experience into a positive one, for example, reflecting on the lessons that their experiences have taught them. They may feel that they have grown in wisdom or sensitivity or somehow become a 'better person' because of their circumstances.

Goffman's theory was developed during the early 1960s and reflects the social values and norms of that time. In contemporary society, it seems that wider range of options is available to stigmatized groups. These include activism and campaigning to transform social attitudes and end discrimination. Examples of this can be seen in the disability rights movement and also in the responses of the gay community, which have challenged society's homophobic attitudes, enabling individuals to come out and find solidarity in the gay pride movement.

Interactionist perspective may be limited in that it does not address the reasons underlying why stigma occurs; it focuses attention on the victim rather than examining the reasons for discrimination against particular groups. Nevertheless, it draws attention to the stress that can accompany stigmatizing experiences, including illness and disability. It also highlights the need for coping strategies in response to the challenges to identity that these experiences may represent. As a consequence, interactionist perspective has had a strong influence on research in medical sociology, much of which is focused on interactions between professionals and patients, and the experiences of people with particular conditions.

The contemporary relevance of sociological perspectives on identity and illness has been emphasized by Mike Bury (1997). Increasing life expectancy and technological advances means that, in contemporary society, an increasing number of people are surviving for a longer period. While growing older does not inevitably lead to poor health, such as a trend is also accompanied by an increasing number of people are likely to find that they cannot sustain the values of independence and achievement that they may have assumed would carry them through adult life.

Not surprisingly, then, the onset of chronic illness may represent a profound threat to personal identity. Bury (1997) illustrates this through the notion of illness as a biographical disruption, illness being not just a physical experience but a social one. It disrupts the pattern of daily life and social relationships. However, illness also creates tasks in relation to maintaining a sense of identity and preserving one's cultural competence in the eyes of others.

## Social Constructionist Perspective and Beyond

So far we have examined perspectives that examine the impact of social processes on the meanings of phenomena such as health and illness. These perspectives suggest that health and illness cannot be understood completely as fixed and unchanging entities. Instead, the meanings attributed to health and illness states may differ at different historical periods and between different cultures. Within Western culture, for example, homosexuality is no longer perceived as a disease. At the same time, new diseases and syndromes, such as 'attention deficit disorder' and 'premenstrual syndrome' describe behaviour that would in previous decades have been understood in very different terms.

Sociologists have also explored the formation of ideas about health and illnesses, examining the role of different groups, such as professionals and scientists, in the production of discourses of health. These debates have implications for the study of lay perspectives, which may differ significantly from scientific and professional views. There has been a general shift away from approaches assuming that medical science is 'right' and other views 'wrong'. This has been accompanied by a shift away from approaches that seek to use sociological knowledge to identify the deficits in lay people's knowledge in order to offer correctives and to increase compliance with medical advice. Instead, there is a growing recognition that professional and lay views are both socially constructed. This means that they cannot easily be categorized as 'right' or 'wrong' because they both arise from the experiences and circumstances of different groups within society.

The writings of Foucault (1976, 1980) have been studied by sociologists seeking to explore further this process of the social constriction of medical knowledge. The notion of the gaze has been used to explain the processes that enabled a medical understanding of the body to emerge during the 18th century. This perspective draws attention to the surveillance and control that are exercised through medical practices. Today, the bodies of the healthy as well as sick people are seen as being increasingly under surveillance. Medical practice is no longer concerned with just the treatment of disease but has been extended into new areas such as prevention and health promotion. These practices, while apparently beneficial, may have negative consequences. While exercising care, health professionals may also be exercising power and control.

## Health and Work Perspectives

A number of theoretical approaches can be utilized in order to understand the effects of work on health:

- The social causation approach seeks to explain the origin of work related-ill health, its social distribution and its impact on different groups. This model is similar to the materialist/structural approach developed by the authors of the Black report (Townsend et al., 1988). It is also the approach adopted by researchers working within a Marxist or political economy perspective.

- The social constructionist perspective is concerned with ideas about risk and hazard. Rather than taking these for granted, social constructionist perspective suggests that our ability to recognize hazards and respond to notions of approach builds on the interactionist perspective in sociology, and some accounts taking this further to suggest that risks and hazards cannot be said to exist in any real sense at all.

One way of understanding the social causation approach is to think in terms of the social and environmental conditions that determine exposure to risk (Eakin and MacEachen, 1998). While risks may be a fact of life, an exposure to risk is not inevitable but arises here from how work is organized. Changes in production processes, such as the introduction of assembly line methods, can affect the pace and nature of work activities, increasing the wear and tear on the body and leading to stress and ill health. From this perspective, questions relating to who makes the decisions and who controls the work processes and activities seem important.

The social causation approach takes as its starting point the need to understand the underlying conditions of the physical environment. Together with social conditions and power relationships, these determine both who is at risk and the degree of risk. This approach offers a dynamic model that can be used to analyse the health effects of recent changes in employment. These have arisen from a number of global trends including a shift in investment and employment from manufacturing to service industries and the growing influence of large multinational corporations.

## Perspectives on Gender

Feminists and feminist studies have all along had grapple with the fact of the material bodies of women in their attempts to find the base for their theories of women's oppression, subordination and exploitation, as well as strategies to overcome the same.

The different discourses the human body has been perceived differently and rather narrowly, as for instance, by Marx as the economic body, by Freud as the sexual body, in scientific and medical discourse as the mechanical body, by modern-day reproductive scientists and biologists as the hormonal body, in population discourse as the fertile body and so on, rather than the body as a whole, constituting an individual (Gupta, 2000).

Feminists brought in another aspect of the medicalization of life by analysing how it related to women specifically. Besides pointing out the medicalization of reproductive processes, they also showed that power did not only pertain to the asymmetrical relations between the doctor and laypersons, but it had to do with the unequal power relations between women and men as (during the time when the critique was first made) the medical professionals (especially gynaecologists) were mostly men (Gupta, 2000). The development and use of reproductive technologies contributes further to the medicalization of life.

For the women's movement to effect a change in unequal gender relations it is important to gain an insight into the sources of power and how it works. The sociology of reproduction is not only about how reproduction is controlled by whom, and for what purpose. It is also about how our knowledge of reproduction has come to be dominated by particular ideologies and views about women prevailing in medical science. Patriarchal control over women's reproduction is closely linked to the control over women's sexuality, the control over women's productive or labour power, property and other economic resources, and control over women's mobility. Therefore, women's strategies for emancipation must embrace all these areas. Patriarchal control over women is linked at a macro level with the economic and political control of people and lands, including political hegemonic interests of certain countries and commercial interests. There are various factors and different actors which play a role: the medical profession and its role in medical control; access to or denial of medical services for fertility control mediated by the medical profession and the state, based on theories of economic development – whether the nation needs more or fewer people (and perhaps what kind of people). Other factors and actors include (organized) religion, the so-called moral guardians of society, population controllers and commercial interests such as those of multinational pharmaceutical companies and commercial providers of technologies which are used for fertility control and management and the media (Gupta, 2000).

Marxists explain gender relations as the outcome of the specific relation between production and reproduction in given context. Reproduction, according to them, refers not only to biological reproduction but to the entire maintenance process that keeps workers functional; it is done mainly in the home, by women. The major Marxist statement on reproductive relations was made by Engels in *The Origin of the Family, Private Property and the State*. But 'the world historical defeat for the female sex' is given no material reproductive substructure, criticizes Mary O'Brien (1981: 143). Even socialist feminists relate the oppression of women to Marxist ideas about exploitation, oppression and labour. Mies (1981: 17) questions the Marxist terminology 'production-reproduction', because production of money is seen as primary and the 'production' of children and life is seen as secondary. According to Marx, 'work' is characterized as a process of 'appropriation of nature' through sensuous, objective activity (Marx and Engels, 1970). Mies observes that as a result of the capitalist division of labour women's role in childbearing and child rearing is falsely characterized as 'nature' and not as 'work'. This is the reconceptualization of women's reproductive work within the Marxist framework. However, women's relationship to nature is not one of the domination but of cooperation with their own bodies and with the earth. Men's self-conception of being human, i.e., productive, is usually linked to the invention and 'control' of tools.

Although the term 'reproduction' is ambiguous and has several levels of meaning, it is used here to mean human biological reproduction. Reproductive processes are far from being mere biological events. They cannot be seen in isolation from social reality and are an important factor in the reproduction of patriarchal relations. The term 'patriarchy' is used here 'to refer to male domination, to the power relationship by which men dominate women, and to characterize a system whereby women are kept subordinate in a number of ways' (Bhasin, 1993: 3). Kamla Bhasin draws on Sylvia Walby's definition. Walby (1990) had pointed out that it is important to understand patriarchy as 'a system of social structures and practices in which men dominate, oppress and exploit women'. This helps us to reject the notion of biological determinism or the notion that every individual man is always in a dominant position and every woman in a subordinate one. Linked to this system is the ideology that men are superior to women, that women are and should be controlled by men and that women are part of men's property (Bhasin, 1993: 3).

Gerda Lerner (1986) proposes that the appropriation and commodification of women's sexual and reproductive capacity by men lay at the foundation of private property, that in fact, it preceded the foundation of private property and class society. Control over one's own reproduction and reproductive freedom concerns all women everywhere in the world, no matter where they live, or what culture, religion or ethnic group they belong to. However, as Petchesky (1980: 667) points out, it is important to keep in mind that 'women's reproductive situation is never the result of biology alone, but of biology mediated by social and cultural organization'.

To one degree or another all the chapters in this volume build on the medicalization and social interactionist model of health. The patriarchy tradition is helpful in explaining the gender inequality in the health. Although the particular subject matter of each chapter is different, however, the women in general are the passive recipient of health care and in turn it reflects the social structure of the society. The different stages in women's life particularly related to health are reflected by understanding the context and particular social structure of the society. It helps in understanding the genesis and direction of the outcome. Beyond this, all the chapters tell us something about the health care issues and the wider society within which that problem is situated.

## References

Bhasin, Kamla (1993), *What is Patriarchy?*, New Delhi: Kali for Women.

Bury, M. (1997), *Health and Illness in a Changing Society*, London: Routledge and Kegan Paul.

Doyal, L. (1979), *The Political Economy of Health*, London: Pluto Press.

Eakin, J. and E. MacEachen (1988), 'Health and the Social Relations of Work: A Study of the Health Related Experiences of Employees in Small Workplaces', *Sociology of Health and Illness*, 20(66): 896–914.

Foster, P. (1995), *Women and the Health Care Industry: An Unhealthy Relationship?*, Buckingham: Open University Press.

Foucault, M. (1976), *The Birth of the Clinic: An Archaeology of Medical Perception*, London: Tavistock.

——. (1980), *The History of Sexuality: An Introduction*, Vol. I, New York: Vintage Books.

Goffman, I. (1963), *Stigma*, London: Penguin.

Gupta, Jyotsna Agnihotri (2000), *New Reproductive Technologies, Women's Health and Autonomy: Freedom or Dependency*, New Delhi: Sage Publications.

Illich, Ivan (1977), *The Limits to Medicine*, Harmondsworth: Penguin.

——. (1975), *Medical Nemesis*, London: Calder and Boyars.

Lerner, Gerda (1986), *The Creation of Patriarchy*, Oxford: Oxford University Press.

Marx, Karl and F. Engels (1970), *The German Ideology*, New York: C.J. Arthur.

McTaggart, L. (1996), *What Doctors Do Not Tell You: The Truth About the Dangers of Modern Medicine*, London: Thornsons.

Mead, George Herbert (1934), *Mind, Self and Society from the Standpoint of Social Behaviorist*, Chicago: Chicago University Press.

Mies, M. (1981), 'Social Origins of the Sexual Division of Labour', Occasional Paper, The Hague: Institute of Social Studies.

Navarro, V. (1979), *Medicine under Capitalism*, London: Croom Helm.

O'Brien, Mary (1981), *The Politics of Reproduction*, London: Routledge and Kegan Paul.

Parsons, Talcott (1951), *The Social System*, London: Routledge and Kegan Paul.

——. (1975), 'The Sick Role and the Role of the Physician Reconsidered', *Milbank Memorial Fund Quarterly*, Vol. 53, No. 3, Summer, pp. 257–78.

Petchesky, R.P. (1980), 'Reproductive Freedom: Beyond 'a Woman's Right to Choose'', *Signs: Journal of Women in Culture and Society*, Special Issue on Women and Sexuality, Vol. 5, No. 4, pp. 661–85.

Townsend, Peter et al. (1988), *Health and Deprivation: Inequality and the North*, London: Routledge.

Walby, S. (1990), *Theorising Patriarchy*, Oxford: Basil Blackwell.

Zola, I. (1972), 'Medicine as an Institution of Social Control', *Sociological Review*, Vol. 20, No. 4, pp. 487–504.

# 2 Gender Inequality

## Perceptive Threat to Health

Impressive achievements and intolerable shortcomings characterize India's health programme over the past fifty years. Not only has there been a decline in mortality rates, but life expectancy and infant survival conditions have also improved. But, it is still very high when we compare with other countries. The World Bank notes that public health financing in India is characterized by an emphasis on hospital, rather than primary care; urban rather than rural population; medical offices rather than paramedics; services that have larger private rather than social returns; and family planning and child health exclusion of wider aspects of female health. In fact, gender differences in health and mortality have not only perpetuated but also accentuated. Therefore, the present chapter will discuss on health as a dimension of discrimination in the social change perspective. The first part will focus on the theoretical perspectives critically analysing the position of women in the process of development. The second part will delineate on: (a) demographic indicators of women's health status; (b) nutritional pattern among women; (c) unequal access to health care; and (d) family planning programmes.

The status of women is a complex issue. It is not amenable to any simplistic explanation of social reality. Literature on the status of women is varied and addresses mainly the key issues affecting the women in various areas of development, such as education, employment, polity, society, law, health, etc. The Constitution of India not only grants equality to women but also empowers the state to adopt measures of positive discrimination in favour of women. Within the framework of a democratic polity, our laws, development policies, plans and programmes have all aimed at women's emancipation. But, the inequalities inherent in traditional structures have still a significant bearing on women in different spheres of life.

The International Conference on Population and Development in Cairo in 1994 placed reproductive health at the centre stage of demographic objective instead of fertility reduction. The Cairo conference recognized women's rights as individual reproductive rights. Gender equity and equality was accepted as a goal for sustained and substantial development. Gender equity and equality; infant, child and maternal mortality reduction; and the provision of universal access to reproductive health services, including family planning services are some of the areas for achieving the gender equity which are necessary to reduce the threat to women's reproductive health.

## I

In this part, we would discuss the various theoretical perspectives ranging from the theory of cultural dualism, social evolutionary theory, idea of developmentalism, dependency theory, biological perspective, Marxian theory, target-group approach and patriarchy approach. These different perspectives and approaches would explain the problems and prospects of women's development.

### Theory of Cultural Dualism

The argument that women are a culturally constructed gender category rather than simply a biological sex led to a much broader feminist challenge to existing knowledge of the relations between men and women. Ortner (1974), in an ambitious attempt to avoid biological determinism while still explaining women's subordination as a universal phenomenon, asked what it was that would lead every culture to place a lower value on women than on men. She concluded that every society made a distinction between nature and culture. Drawing on the work of Simone de Beauvoir (1952) and Nancy Chodorow (1978), she argued that women's social ties to children through pregnancy and breast-feeding ensured that women appeared to be closer to nature than men. Simone de

Beauvoir is one of the chief protagonists of cultural dualism. It is based on the perception that the secondary status of women is universalistic. She tries to locate the origins of women's subordination in part, in her relationship to nature and nature's relationship to culture. Man controls nature through culture, so he is superior to both nature and woman. Elaborating the perspective of cultural dualism, Whyte and Whyte (1982) argue that what is certain is that today it is very difficult for women to manifest at the same time their autonomous individuality and their feminine destiny. They also suggest that the western woman seeks liberation as an individual, while the Asian woman seeks greater satisfaction by the improvement of her family's economic situation and of her status within the family. The primary role of the woman is always manifested in her family. The society at large views their economic role as secondary so that they are pushed out of the market. Though the theory of cultural dualism lacks coherence, it provides a useful analysis by supporting a sophisticated view of the internal dynamics of culture as it relates to the position of women.

## Social Evolutionary Theory

Social evolutionary theory is preoccupied with the question as to whether women's position is becoming better or worse as societies undergo change. By giving emphasis on the division of labour, social evolutionary theory provides an explanation for inequality within societies. With specialization each labouring group becomes more efficient thereby creating a base for larger productivity. Generally speaking, societies seeking a higher level of productivity are expected to move toward greater specialization (Parsons, 1966: 47). Therefore, simple societies with less differentiation among social units are less productive and poor. Within complex industrialized societies these groups who perform less specialized roles are less productive and earn lower incomes. This explanation of inequality has been the premise of a great deal of scholarly work on sexual inequality, particularly among economists. However, feminist scholars like Easter Boserup have questioned the linkage between specialization, technology and rewards. Boserup demonstrates that women have been relegated to jobs in the relatively unimportant sectors of the economy involving low level of specialization, because they fall on the lower side of the 'productivity gap' and therefore suffer inequality (Boserup, 1970: 65–68). Social differentiation has a similar effect on the participation of women in public life. This increased the gap between domestic and external arenas, and women are relegated to be more particularistic concerns of domestic life. With this, they seem to have lost the opportunity to participate in decision-making in the public domain. Thus, with the growth of highly industrialized complex societies, one observes the domestication of women, which in turn lowers their status.

## Developmentalism

The perception that modernization has had differential effects on men and women has led planners to seek to describe the obstacles preventing women from participating in development. The United Nations Conference on Women, held in Mexico City, in 1975, focused worldwide attention on the need for 'intensified action to ensure the full integration of women in the development process' (United Nations, 1975). The developmentalism perspective presented at the UN conference has three notions about social change that differ from the assumption of conventional modernization theory: (a) changes introduced in one sector may not generate compatible changes in various other sectors of society; (b) there are always contradictions in the process of social change; and (c) national elites and external forces play major role in ushering in programmes aimed at social change favouring women. Failures in implementation have led revisionist developmentalists to consider decision-making by individuals as well as governments.

## Dependency Theory

Dependency theory focuses attention on constraints placed on development by international forces. It gained some currency as modernization theorists had difficulty in explaining in Third World countries. Dependency theory attempts to locate systematic connections among the contradictions noted by developmentalists by pursuing the linkages through the socio-economic infrastructures of the countries concerned. Although the phase of colonialism was over, advanced nations held economic hegemony through controls of markets and superior technology. One consequence of such a strategy was the priority given to heavy industry, urban growth and export-oriented commercial crops, leaving the backward rural sector in status quo (Inkeles and Smith, 1974). Another variant of dependency theory as it relates directly to women was conceptualized by Marxist feminists with an international orientation. For them, the model of patriarchy rooted in the mode of production is part of an international system based on dependency occupies a central place. Capitalism in different countries has been dislodging working women for agriculture at a fast rate, but without providing opportunities for their absorption in industry. Therefore, female labour force participation in developing countries has declined with development. Women hold a disproportionate number of jobs in the informal sector, particularly the low status ones like domestic servants, street vendors, etc.

## Biological Perspective

Perhaps the most influential and controversial theory of the emergence of gender identity is that of Sigmund Freud. According to him, the learning of gender differences in infants and young children is centred on possession or absence of male sexual organs. Freud is careful to say that it is not just the anatomical distinctions that matter but possession or absence of male sexual organs is symbolic of masculinity and femininity. Physical differences between a man and a woman become the basis of building a system of reciprocal roles and in the process the wife's role, including the nurturing, subordinated while the economic functions of man were defined as superior and superordinate and boys and girls are socialized to fulfil the roles. However, the division of roles between the sexes has its origin in the biologically different functions of males and females. But this does not mean that man is biologically the more active. In the words of Linton, 'all societies prescribed different attitudes and activities to men and to women. Most of them try to rationalize these prescriptions in terms of their physiological differences between the sexes and their roles in reproduction. However, a comparative study of the statuses ascribed to man and woman in different cultures seems to show that while such factors have served as starting for the development of a division of actual ascription are almost entirely determined by culture'.

### Marxian Perspective

Marx has not exclusively dealt with the theory of woman's emancipation. Of course, one finds new references in the works of Marx about family, about changing sex relations and about women's participation in the capitalist production process. Marx has noticed the importance of the female as an economic production unit in the social organization of society until the capitalist (bourgeoisie) society came into being. In the *Communist Manifesto,* he and Engels predict the dissolution of not only the family in its old form but all pre-capitalist forms of exploitation and oppression and visualize those who have no access to the means of production will be ruled by the laws of motion. Engels (1970) traced the link between the rise of private property, monogamy, patriarchal family and the state. This was an attempt to show the origin of subordination of women by men and based on that locating determination of woman's subordination analytically. Engels presents historical process by which a woman is transformed from free-equal productive member of the society to subordinate and dependent wife.

### Target Group Approach

The target group approach is based on the assumption that disadvantaged sections of society need special programmes for their advancement. In the intermediate decades after independence little or no effort was made by the planners in developing countries to integrate women into development plans. Development plans made provisions for industrialization, rural development, education and health programmes, etc. Barbara Rogers (1980) has carried out a comprehensive analysis of how the orientations of development planners affect the role of Third World women. She shows how neo-colonialism and multilateralism have further reduced the access to and control over nature. Special programmes should be designed and targeted for specific groups like women. Boserup and others also point out that failure to give full access to women in employment actually defeats national development plans in a number of ways, and where improvements did not occur for women, the problem was seen to be consequence of imperfect integration of women into development.

Corresponding to this is the debate on the relationship between sexual equality and socio-economic inequalities in stratified societies. In case of India, these studies have been done to bring out the increasingly adverse impact of the processes of change on women. The macro-indicators include the adverse decline in the sex ratio, the differentials in morality, literacy access to health care and decline in women's education (Mazumdar, 1979). Responding to these concerns, the Indian planners have been attempting to design new policy instruments for women's development. These are basically target group-oriented and attempt to provide for the diversification and expansion of opportunities for education and training of women, provision of credit facilities for self-employment and small sector employment programmes for women.

## Patriarchy

The word 'patriarchy' literally means the rule of the father or the 'patriarch', and originally it was used to describe a specific type of 'male-dominated family'. This refers to the power relationships by which men dominate women, and to characterize a system whereby women are kept subordinate in a number of ways (Bhasin, 1993). The conception of patriarchy as universal is logically based on the conception of woman as a universal category. Whether or not women are explicitly conceived of as a class whose interests are opposed to those of men as a class (a position taken, for example, by Firestone, 1979) and Millett (1977), men are seen as having and defending power over women.

Thus, patriarchy has been used by feminist scholars as a theoretical construct to explain the structure underlying the subordination of women and as one hindering the development of women. The structure of the patriarchal system has been conceived at psychological, cultural and material levels (Mazumdar, 1979). The centrality of the family (which is a primary unit) as an entity in which the productivity activities are undertaken. This unit in which the production and reproduction of social life is carried on has definitely a major role in the development of women. Women's experience within the household varies by class, ethnic group, caste, culture and religion. It is thus necessary to explore the differing principles and notions of family and kinship. It is the notions of family and kinship that shape the woman's position in the society. The process of socialization starts from this basic social unit, i.e., the family (Mitra, Pathak and Mukherji, 1980). So, here starts the process of subordination.

Besides the above theoretical explanations of women's subordination at global level and in the Indian society, the roles women play in the society and the images that have developed of them, are not simply from exigencies of biology and social situations, but are rather deeply rooted in the myths, legends, religion and culture. Therefore, it is here that one observes the underlying causes that keep woman in subservience as 'second sex' devoid of any identity. This tradition has gained much significance and with the passage of time came to be accepted as the unwritten law of the land. Moreover, the demographic indicators like mortality rate, infant mortality rate, life expectancy, reproductive diseases, etc., will all able to spell out the prevailing inequality among males and females.

A theoretical approach to the problems and prospects of women's development is extremely essential to have a thorough understanding of the subject. Laws by themselves cannot bring social change. We need to understand the social values, social structure and the role of the productive process. One assumption to all the perspectives is that the position of women has not registered significant improvement despite the efforts at modernization.

## II

Keeping in view the different theoretical perspectives that we have discussed in the preceding section, we would like to analyse the empirical facts to understand the gender discrimination in the context of the health problem. This section deals mainly demographic indicators, nutritional pattern, unequal access to health care, and women and family planning.

### Demographic Indicators

Although there has been an overall improvement in the health conditions of both males and females, but women still get differentiated from men when it comes to providing medical care and this shows comparative low status of women in our society. According to UNICEF, 12 million girls are born in India every year, out of which 25 per cent do not survive beyond the 15th year. The reason behind this is that the mortality rate of 0–5 years age group is about 20 times greater than any other age group. Female mortality rate up to the age of 40 years is higher than the rate for mortality, as a whole. Although an increase in the life expectancy for women has been recorded in absolute numbers, but in comparison to the life expectancy of males, it is still lower. Strikingly, maternal mortality rates are particularly high (Padmanabha, 1982). Even the number of years they stay healthy is much lesser.

The most populations in the world the sex ratio at birth tends to be favourable to females even though the males outnumber them at younger ages due to slightly more males being born than females (the sex ratio at birth varies between 102 to 107 boys per 100 girls for biological reasons), but this advantage of males get neutralized by about the age of 20 due to higher mortality among boys than girls (Premi, 2001). In India, and in few other countries of South Asia and West Asia, the situation is different due to neglect of females at almost all ages. In the absence of hard data on Sample Registration of Birth (SRB) particularly from the Civil Registration System, we had been assuming 105 male births for every 100 female births for almost half a century. We have also assumed that the same has remained constant over time. There has, however, been a possibility that SRB has changed over time in favour of females. The Sample Registration System (SRS)-based sex ratio at birth over the 1981–90 period was 109.5 male births per 100 female births. SRS data for the 1990s indicates further imbalance in SRB, it being 111 male births for every 100 female births.

At the national level, the child sex ratio (in population aged 0–6 years) declined from 962 in 1981 to 945 in 1991. In the 2001 Census child sex ratio had declined further by 18 points from a 945 in 1991 to 927 in 2001. Even, in the provisional 2011 Census report, it has further dropped to 914, which is the lowest since independence.

In examining child sex ratio, one should, however concentrate on infant and child mortality since they affect the child survival most. At the national level there have been only a few years when infant mortality for females has been lower than males but it has been mostly higher. For example, between 1995 and 1999, the female IMR has been higher by a couple of points than male IMR (1995: male 73, female 76; 1996: male 71, female 73; 1997: male 70, female 72; 1998: male 70, female 73; 1999: male 69.8, female 70.8). The female age-specific death rates (ASDRs) for the age group 0–4 and 5–9 years have also remained higher all the years from 1984 to 1998 (1984 – male 39.6, female; 1998 – male 21.0, female 24.1) (Registrar General of India 1999; *SRS Bulletin*, April 2001). It is noteworthy that the 1984–1990 data relate to the period when children aged 0–6 years counted in 1991 Census were born. Similarly, the data for the period 1994–1999 relate to the period when children aged 1–6 years were born (Premi, 2001). It is due to pathological reasons that high morbidity and low nutritional status. Girls tend to be brought for treatment at more critical stages of illness or are taken to less qualified doctors, so their mortality even under treatment is likely to be greater. The higher mortality of girls under 0–6 is largely responsible for the skewed sex ratio. Mathur (1985) opined that at birth chances of survival for a male child are less than those for a female child but after the neo-natal stage, social factors such as care, immunization, nutrition of the mother and child, and sanitation come into force and govern the survival prospects of an infant.

Ghosh (1985) is also of the view that the adverse sex ratio in our country is mainly because of high risk of female deaths from infancy to the end of the reproductive period. The same neglect is evident in exceedingly high maternal mortality rates, mainly because health care workers are in attendance for fewer than half the births. Mitra (1979), for the first time in 1974, gave a warning that the continuous decline in sex ratio of female to male would threaten the very survival of the female sex in India. He described Indian women as a 'declining sex'. The increased sex ratio of the population during the 1980s was concentrated heavily amongst children. The data suggests that over a million additional girls went 'missing' between 1981 and 1991 that is over and above the numbers already implied missing by the skewed sex ratios of 1981 (Gupta and Bhat, 1997). Meanwhile, both the sex ratio and child mortality have remained constant, suggesting that most of this may be attributable to the practice of sex-selective abortion or unreported infanticide. Excess female child mortality after birth continues to be the dominant practice in remaining female children in India. The rough estimates for 1981–91 indicate that there were perhaps four times as many excess female child deaths taking place after birth than before birth or as unreported infanticides. The sex ratio is adverse for women among all religious groups, and in both rural and urban areas. Even in the richest states of India (e.g., Haryana and Punjab), it is extremely adverse for women. The only region where the sex ratio is favourable for women is Kerala where the literacy for women is also the highest in India.

Lack of widespread availability of safe abortion services also has adverse impact on women's health. According to some estimates, roughly 5 million abortions are performed annually in India, the large majority (about 4.5 million) illegally (Khan et al., 1993; UNICEF, 1990; cited in Jejeebhoy, 1995). As a result, abortion-related mortality and morbidity continue to be high with at least 10 per cent of all maternal deaths resulting from abortion. Although, since 1972, abortion has been made legal and officials claim that pregnancy termination services are widely available, but in actual practice the situation is different. In 1981, of the 62,000 physicians trained to perform abortion, only 1,600 were working in rural areas and only 10 per cent of rural health centres were equipped for pregnancy (Conly and Camp, 1992).

Gender inequality also persists among the elderly women. There have been improvements in women's life expectancy relative to men's. An Indian woman now lives 18 years longer than four decades ago. In the year 1970, life expectancy at birth for women was 49.1 years which by 2000 increased to 62.9 years and by 2010 67.5 years. As a consequence of this and other socio-cultural reasons, more women tend to be widowed than men; for example, in 1988 nearly two-thirds of Indian elderly women were widowed compared to about a fifth of the men (NSSO, 1991). This happens due to several reasons in general. First, women tend to be younger than their husbands and cultural and social norms inhibit them from remarriage. Second, the problem of elderly women in the female population is currently greater than the corresponding proportion of elderly man. In addition, the rate at which the female population is ageing is faster than that of male (Sharma and Xenos, 1992).

Ageing is often perceived as a deterioration in health. Most research and services tend to concentrate on women of reproductive age ignoring those beyond these years. While the process of growing old may bring some improvements and benefits to a woman in the post-middle age period, these may diminish as she advances into old age or when she is widowed (Rao and Townsend, 1999). A woman often derives power from authority from her association with the male head of family. If this association suffers an erosion, her access to resources for care and sustenance is reduced, making her vulnerable. The risk increases for women who have no assets for survival such as education, possessions or social status. This vulnerability may be compounded by failing health and disability. Thus, an indigent and physically frail, elderly widow is the most defenceless in the Indian context (Chen and Dreze, 1995). It is important to note that the elderly women suffer not only from ailments specific to ageing, but also from ill health accumulated over the life cycle which may manifest in old age in an aggravated form. The proportion of women reporting 'problem of joints' is higher than that of men. This is expected, as after menopause women are particularly prone to the development of osteoarthritis, a painful degenerative joint disease (Tinker et al., 1994). Disability also affects the health of elderly people. It is well known that the prevalence of blindness in India varies not only by geographical location and degree of urbanization, but also by gender (World Bank, 1944). The National Family Health Survey found that the prevalence of partial blindness was 2,839 per 100,000 for women of all ages and 2,346 per 100,000 for men of all ages (IIPS, 1995). Reasons for this gender pattern could be partly biological and partly behavioural. Disorders during pregnancy can cause cataract, while diabetes, glaucoma and metabolic disorders can also increase the risk of cataract.

Several health conditions affecting elderly women such as changes in the skeletal, cardiovascular, nervous, skin, genitourinary and gastro-intestinal systems are caused by declines in ovarian hormonal levels triggered by menopause. Due to the absence of ovarian steroids, chronic diseases such as osteoporosis, coronary heart disease and cerebrovascular develop (Tinker et al., 1994). Gynaecological cancers, prolapse and fistulae are some conditions afflicting the elderly women and are the result of early child and high fertility. Elderly women may find it difficult to disclose to younger members the nature of their illness, especially if these are gynaecological problems. This is one reason why conditions such as prolapse tend to be neglected.

However, as is true of most self-reported morbidity, it is difficult to distinguish from the data whether the differences between men and women are due to variations in illness perception and reporting or in gender-based biological burdens. More research is needed before any conclusion can be drawn on morbidity patterns. In the absence of data for disease-wise mortality between male and females in elderly group, the death differentials could be because of susceptibility to diseases, differing exposure to risk, differential utilization of health services or differential reporting.

## Nutritional Pattern

In Indian society poor nutrition is caused not only by lack of food or poverty but there are also many socio-cultural factors which are responsible for this. Today, India is in the bottom of world's maiden nutrition barometer, announced by 'Save the Children' recently. The report says that children in poor households are more than twice as likely to be stunted as those in affluent ones.

Optimum standard of nutrition is determined on the basis of body weight, sex, climate and nature of the work performed. More than half of the women in India do not get the recommended dietary intake of nutrients (Kulkarni, n.d.). Generally, the poor nutritional status of Indian girls and women is part of a vicious cycle that has particularly devastating consequences for pregnant and lactating women and their infants. Malnourished women are more likely to give birth to low birth weight babies, and if the underweight baby is a female who survives, she in turn is likely to continue to be undernourished throughout her childhood, adolescence and adult life. This lack of nourishment has also detrimental effects on her reproductive and lactating capacities.

In India, all nutritional programmes are directed towards the needs of pregnant and lactating mothers. However, in spite of these, there is nutritional deficiency in women starting from infancy to pregnancy and than again after crossing the childbearing age. It cannot be denied that poverty is a major cause of malnutrition and undernourishment. But its more unfavourable impact on women's nutritional standards shows the connivance of poverty and socio-cultural values operative among them. Poor nutrition of girls, especially in childhood and adolescence, has serious consequences (Jejeebhoy, 1995). Anaemia is a major health problem among Indian women. Studies carried out by the Indian Council of Medical Research found that over 65 per cent of girls aged 1–14 surveyed in the cities of Hyderabad, New Delhi, and Calcutta were anaemic (ICMR, 1982). Anaemia is particularly widespread among women during pregnancy, when iron requirement increases nearly fivefold (Hallberg, 1988). A variety of studies have shown that a high percentage of pregnant women in India are anaemic, particularly in the last trimester. One study conducted in the rural districts of Gujarat and Maharashtra found that about 90 per cent of pregnant women suffered from anaemia. Other studies have also found rates of anaemia between 50 and 90 per cent among pregnant women (Sheshadari and Gopaldas, 1989; Raman, 1980, 1988, Agarwal, Agarwal and Tripathi, 1987; Agarwal, 1984). A recent population-based survey of pregnant women showed some degree of anaemia and that 56 per cent had severe anaemia. An analysis of the data from the referral hospital for the area revealed that severe anaemia contributed, directly or indirectly, to 35 per cent of all in-hospital maternal deaths (Sarin, 1995). Even, the above referred 'Save the Children' report indicates the almost half of Indian children are underweight and stunted, and over 70 per cent of women and kids have serious nutritional deficiencies, such as anaemia.

Poor nutrition becomes evident among females during infancy, persists through childhood, and tends to increase with age. In a study of two Delhi slum populations, Basu (1989) found that only 50–65 per cent of female infants below the age of one year received adequate nourishment or were only mildly malnourished. For female children aged 5–9, the percentage fell to about 30–35. It is probable that the result of this anthropometric study reflects not only differential nutrition but also differential morbidity. The NNMB surveys (1980) documented low intakes of Vitamin A and iron among girl children and adolescents. Vitamin A deficiency, which has been firmly linked to high mortality and morbidity in children, is likely to be an underlying cause of high levels of respiratory and genitourinary tract infections in women.

Among many Indian families, the largest share of food is usually given to the bread earner, the next to boys, to the old or sick and the last, to young girls and women in the household (Nagla, 1999). Girls are often neglected in matters of feeding and health care. Discrimination in feeding may begin soon after birth as girls are breastfed less frequently as for shorter duration than boys. In recent years, increasing attention has been given to differentials in the allocation of food within households. However, rates of malnutrition among children and women are high. Ethnographic literature suggests that females are not fed as well, as males in northern India (Harriss, 1966; Miller, 1981). Studies in Uttar

Pradesh (Khan and others, 1989), Andhra Pradesh (Bidinger, Nag and Babu, 1986) and Tamil Nadu (Devadas and Kamalanthan, 1985) all indicate that female children are discriminated against when it comes to the allocation of food within households. Marked differences exist between what is fed to boys and girls. The discrepancy increases with age. According to figures obtained from the National Nutrition Monitoring Bureau (NNMB), in the age group of 10–15 years, boys are fed 31 gm of pulses a day, whereas girls get only 25 gm a day. Boys get more of leafy vegetables, more of fruits and more of calcium. As children grow up and take up a sedentary or active job, the gap in the degrees of nutrition widens even more. For instance, a woman in a sedentary job get 403 gm of cereals a day. A man in a similar job gets 475 gm (NNMB, 1980).

The malnutrition prevalent in a significant proportion of adult Indian women can be attributed primarily to inadequate food intake. The households that have theoretically enough food, but the way it is distributed may leave women inadequately nourished. Typically, adult men and male children are fed first. Women eat only after the men have finished, and a young wife must allow her mother-in-law to eat first. Whatever is left is divided among the young mother and her female children (Caldwell, Reddy and Caldwell, 1989; Jeffery, Jeffery and Lyon, 1989). This disparity in the distribution of food may be as much a matter of poor communication as of deliberate practice, since men are normally unaware of how much women eat. Whatever the reason, and given the nutritional demands of child bearing and lactation, the lack of nourishment puts women at particular risk during their child-bearing years. Indian women may be malnourished because of the poor nutritive quality of what is available even when they food.

### Unequal Access to Health Care

Medical and health services too are not evenly available to men and women. For every three men who avail facilities of medical institutions, only one woman does so. This is not because of greater 'healthiness' in women but due to low importance accorded to women's ailments. Women are not only neglected by others, but they also neglect themselves. Fewer women declare themselves ill as compared to men.

A young paediatrician in a Jammu hospital came across a patient, a girl about five years, who had lost a lot of blood in an accident. The girl had to be given blood immediately. The doctor approached the girl's father and asked him to donate a unit of blood as his blood group matched her's. The father was reluctant. '*Yeh to paraya dhan hai. Iske liye mai apni sehat kyun kharab karun?* (She is to go away after her marriage. Why should I harm my health for her?),' he said. Even after a lot of persuasion, he did not relent and walked away. The doctor was stunned. The girl, it was learnt, died a few days later (Srivastava, 2000).

Access to health care is determined by 'need', 'permission', 'ability' and 'availability' (Chatterjee, 1990). Use of health system is determined by perceived need and often 'need' is limited to the childbearing years. Even in the childbearing years use tends to be limited. For example, the NFHS reported that of during the births which occurred in the previous four years, 62 per cent of mothers had received anti-natal care while 26 per cent had delivered in medical institutions and 34 per cent were delivered by trained medical persons (IIPS, 1995). The reason for such low levels of use is that, often women perceive the services of hospitals to be unnecessary. Social and economic norms determine 'permission' and 'ability'. Often women need permission to seek health care. When there is dependence, either physical or financial, on care givers, access is determined by the willingness and ability of the care givers to provide treatment. For example, women who needed treatment for visual disability if they had no sons or could not find alternative escorts (World Bank, 1944). Permission/ability depends upon the geographical proximity and one's purchasing capacity.

There is considerable evidence that male children receive more and better health care at an earlier age than female children do. At the All India Institute of Medical Sciences (AIIMS), New Delhi, of all the surgeries which are conducted on children and infants, 70 per cent are on boys and only 30 per cent on girls. From 1986 to 1999, the number of neo-natal surgeries carried out in intensive care were 2,089. Of these, 1,441 were boys and 648 were girls. On an average, in these 15 years, around 69 per cent of the surgeries were conducted on boys. In 1998, as compared to 117 boys operated in intensive care, only 57 girls were operated. In 1999, of the total 152 surgeries in this category, only 47 were girls. On an average, the same number of boys and girls fall ill and develop complications post birth. But, as compared to boys, less than half the number of girls are brought to hospitals. It may be because when a child has to undergo surgery, the entire family gets involved. Such sufferers are almost always major and also involve expenditure. Though treatment may be free, there are several overhead costs in surgery. This require longer hospitalization and for a family from outside Delhi, this also involves the cost of living in the city (Srivastava, 2000). One study in the Ludhiana district of Punjab found that low-caste female children under age three received less medical care than other children and that the medical care provided tended to be of poorer quality. Two decades later, Das Gupta (1987) found that the situation had not changed. A study in a Ludhiana hospital concluded that gender bias prevented three out of four girls who were ill enough to require hospitalization from receiving the care they needed (Booth and Verma, 1992). Caldwell, Reddy and Caldwell (1983) found that in rural Karnataka, twice as many boys as girls were brought to the primary health centre. And, in a study of one rural area in western Uttar Pradesh, Khan and others (1989) reported that over a one week period roughly three times as many boys as girls were brought to the primary health centre. Seventy-three per cent of male children, compared with 62 per cent of female children, were taken to a health provider or health facility in the event of an acute respiratory infection. For India, as a whole, in 1992–93 more boys than girls were vaccinated and treated for acute respiratory infections and fevers (IIPS, 1995).

Like female children, adult women are also at disadvantageous position with respect to health care. Household surveys typically report more incidence of illness for females than for males (Khan and others, 1989). This finding is especially striking because female morbidity is likely to be underreported for several reasons: women respondents may be reluctant to reveal details of their illnesses to interviewers; they may purposely downplay any health problem to avoid disrupting domestic duties; or, consistent with their socialization, they may not wish to imply that they are asking for medical care. Community-based studies make it clear, however, that one reason for the relatively high morbidity rates among women is that they receive less medical treatment than men (Kielmann and Taylor, 1983; Dandekar, 1975). Hospital and health centre records provide supporting evidence: fewer women than men are hospitalized or visit clinics (Khan and others, 1989; Murthy, 1982). Community-based studies also reveal that a high proportion of women receive no treatment at all for their illnesses and that among those who do, self-care, home remedies and the traditional medical care are the most common methods used. Men are more likely to receive modern medical treatment including high-quality institutional care (Das, Dhanoa and Cowan, 1982; Miller, 1981).

In addition, our health care system is institution-based rather than domicilliary. This generates inhibitions among the rural population about the alien environment of the hospital. Moreover, women are burdened with greater disabilities than men. They have paucity of time, monetary resources and child care facilities. Mobility of women is far more restricted than that of men. Thus, they are deprived of utilization of facilities rendered by the health care system.

Government has been giving a low priority to health sector, which is evident from its various plan outlays. Moreover, inadequate coverage of rural health through primary health centres (PHCs) and non-utilization of the existing PHCs also contribute a lot. Only 50 per cent pregnant women receive antenatal care. Tetanus immunization is done only to 20 per cent pregnant women and still many deliveries are performed through untrained and unskilled midwives. Health care should be a right of every individual and not a privilege. India spends relatively heavily on health both as a percentage of gross domestic product as well as in absolute US dollars terms, when compared to some other countries of the Asian region (Jeffery, Jeffery and Lyon, 1989), yet women remain deprived and marginalized from its ambit. India's spending on health in Twelfth Plan will be 1.67 per cent of its GDP.

## Women and Family Planning

Increasing population is the country's most urgent and pressing problem today, and root of all social and economic ills. The population control programme is, therefore, seen as the panacea for all ills, which will bring down the birth rate through adoption of the small family norm. However, the family planning programmes are overwhelmingly aimed at women. When the policies are framed for control of population, the mention of women appeared. This concern for a reduction in the birth rate flows directly from the theory that population growth is a hinderance to development – a conviction that is maintained despite lack of evidence that such a cause and effect connection exists at all (Krishnaraj, Sudarshan and Shariff, 1999). This has consequences for women. A conceptualization that regards the control of population as a primary objective will not regard women's interests as important. A perception of development as economic growth will forget that development is meant for people and that women are also people. They are simultaneously the means and the ends. As women bear children, fertility reduction implies that women must give birth to fewer babies. The problem is, therefore, seen as one of women's reproductive capacity, and not of social organizations. How is fertility to be curtailed? It can be achieved by curtailing the reproductive capacity of women's bodies directly or by men taking care to prevent impregnation.

Birth control is an important instrument of emancipation for women, but there is a perceptible difference in consequences for women when birth control is imposed, or when the means to do so are unavailable, or the means made are hazardous to life and health. In all such cases, women's power is limited. Fertility control can be liberating only when it consists in not just control of it, but when it implies self-regulation done freely by women.

Since 1970, the use of modern contraceptive methods has risen from about 10 per cent to 40 per cent. Again, the figures vary widely by state, from 53 per cent in Maharashtra to 20 per cent in Uttar Pradesh and Bihar.

The practice of family planning is heavily dominated by sterilization, with over 75 per cent users of modern contraception being sterilized. However, male sterilization accounts for only 10 per cent of all sterilizations while only 7 per cent of couples use condoms (NFHS, 1992–93). Ironically, several medical technologies for family planning have resulted in opposite effect. The burden and responsibility of birth control has been placed on women and specifically on poor women. The family planning technologies like IUDs, tubule legation, indictable contraceptives and laparoscopic tubectomies require professionals to instal them and needs follow-up also. But they hardly get time for follow-up. Moreover, these devices have to be applied by highly trained and experienced hands and within an environment where sterile conditions and adequate aftercare are scrupulously maintained. Most of the times, these technologies have side effects as in the case with injectable and intra-uterine devices. The women suffer from excessive bleeding, cramps, backaches, headaches, dizziness and swelling, etc. (Shramshakti, 1988). Abortion is often denied unless the women coming to family planning centres are made guinea pigs or are forced to participate in trials of experimental contraceptives. Sterilization is being adopted en mass as a method without acknowledging the adverse effects on women who have to resume heavy manual labour soon after. Thus, the inadequacies of health care system at the operational level have rendered unscrupulous many existing methods, which could otherwise be safely promoted.

The most striking aspect of contraceptive use in India is the predominance of sterilization, which accounts for more than 85 per cent of total modern contraceptive use. Female sterilization accounts for 90 per cent of sterilizations (World Bank, 1996). The lack of knowledge about and access to other contraceptive methods reflects the family welfare programme's historical emphasis on sterilization. Increasing contraceptive choice, particularly temporary methods for delaying and spacing pregnancies, is now seen as a high priority.

In India, fertility reduction has been achieved mostly by terminal methods. In the state of Kerala contraceptive practice is almost entirely achieved by women and that too almost entirely through tubectomies. Here comes a paradox. The action is by women apparently because they have had social development and yet it is not liberating for in order that it be liberating women need the possibility of choice of a wide range of methods. If the methods made available are limited and women cannot control them and have to depend on medical staff, to that extent there is less autonomy. Another aspect is the issue of men's responsibility for contraception (Krishnaraj, Sudarshan and Shariff, 1999). Should the onus of birth control be entirely on women, when men are equally responsible for reproduction? Many organizations are demanding this particularly in the context of AIDS (ARROW, 1996). While the dominant ideology of gender relations that regards men as economic providers and women as child bearers and rearers persists in society, this is also reflected among the predominantly male policy makers and health personnel. The state becomes an additional agent for control over women's bodies (Krishnaraj, Sudarshan and Shariff, 1999).

The family welfare programmes rely mainly on women as clients. The advent and proliferation of advanced techniques for sex determination of foetuses like amniocentesis, super sonography, etc., have further aggravated the risk of test of restricting further female population of India.

## Conclusion

The theoretical perspectives explain the unequal position of women either due to patriarchal structure, biological phenomenon, differential development, dependency on men, etc. Besides these, the role women play in a particular society and the images they develop are not simply from exigencies of biology, development and social situations, but are rather deeply rooted in the myths, legends, religion and culture.

The demographic situation of India is averse to the females. Excess female child mortality after birth continues to be the dominant practice in removing female children. Sex-selective abortion is also accounted for gender bias and making sex ratio unfavourable to women. Early marriage and more number of pregnancies result in higher maternal mortality rates. Nutrition is an important element in preserving health. Within households, women and girls are often discriminated against in food allocation. This type of discrimination starts from child birth, with male baby being nursed for longer duration than baby girls and continues over the lifetime. Adolescence is the period of the growth and girls get less than the required daily allowance of nutrients; as a result of this they do not achieve their growth potential causing risks during the critical childbearing years. In the old age also women bear the burden of malnutrition that started very early in life. Also, in time of food shortages, elderly women are most likely to be more affected.

Women of all ages have not only poor access to the health care system but are also less likely to use it. Gender bias in accessing and using health care starts early in life. More boys are brought to clinics for treatment than girls. Girls are provided with poorer medical care. This type of gender discrimination continues in later life as well, where women may downplay their morbidities, attempt home remedies and seek traditional medical treatment before reaching the hospital. Health care utilization behaviour of elderly women will also continue when the pattern is set up in childhood.

Further, the blatant targeting of women in family planning programmes has also adversely affected their health. The lack of information and availability of different family planning methods has its bearing on women's health. If the methods of family planning are limited and women cannot control them, they have to depend on medical staff. Disproportionate emphasis on female sterilization, in conjunction with a lack of concern about health outcomes for women, is a manifestation of gender inequality built in the state government programmes as well as into Indian society.

## References


Agarwal, D.K., K.N. Agarwal and A.M. Tripathi (1987), 'Nutritional Status in Rural Pregnant Women of Bihar and Uttar Pradesh', *Indian Paediatrics*, Vol. 24, No. 2, pp. 119–26.

Agarwal, Kailash N. (1984), 'The Effects of Maternal Iron Deficiency on the Placenta and Foetus', in D.B. Jelliffe and E.F.P. Jelliffe (eds), *Advances in International Maternal and Child Health*, Vol. 4, London: Oxford University Press.

ARROW (1996), *Men's Roles and Responsibilities in Reproduction*, Vol. 2, No. 1, May.

Basu, Alka (1989), 'Is Discrimination in Food Really Necessary for Explaining Sex Differentials in Childhood Mortality?', *Population Studies*, Vol. 43, No. 2, pp. 93–210.

Bidinger, Patricia, M. Nag and P. Babu (1986), *Factors Affecting Intra-Family Food Distribution in a South Indian Village*, New York: Ford Foundation.

Bhasin, Kamla (1993), *What is Patriarchy?* Delhi: Kali for Women.

Booth, Beverley and M. Verma (1992), 'Decreased Access to Medical Care for Girls in Punjab, India: The Roles of Age, Religion, and Distance', *American Journal of Public Health*, Vol. 82, No. 2, pp. 1155–57.

Boserup, Ester (1970), *Women's Role in Economic Development*, London: Allen and Unwin.

Caldwell, J.C., P.H. Reddy and P. Caldwell (1983), 'The Causes of Marriage Change in South India', *Population Studies*, Vol. 37, No. 3, pp. 343–61.

Census of India (2001), *SRS Bulletin*, Vol. 35, No. 1, New Delhi: Registrar General.

Chatterjee, Meera (1990), 'Indian Women: Their Health and Economic Productivity', World Bank Discussion Papers No. 109, Washington, DC: World Bank.

Chodorow, Nancy (1978), *The Reproduction of Mothering: Psychoanalysis and the Sociology of Gender*, Berkeley: University of California Press.

Chen, Martha Alter and Jean Dreze (1995), 'Widowhood and Well-being in Rural North-India', in Monica Das Gupta, Lincoln C. Chen and T.N. Krishnan (eds), *Women's Health in India: Risk and Vulnerability*, Bombay: Oxford University Press.

Conly, Shanti R. and Sharon L. Camp (1992), *India's Family Planning Challenge: From Rhetoric to Action*, Washington, DC: The Population Crisis Committee.

Dandekar, K. (1975), 'Has the Proportion of Women in India's Population been Declining?', *Economic and Political Weekly*, Vol. 10, No. 42.

Das Gupta, Monica (1987), 'Selective Discrimination against Female Children in Rural Punjab, India', *Population and Development Review*, Vol. 13, No. 1, pp. 77–100.

Das Gupta, Monica and P.N. Mari Bhat (1997), 'Fertility Decline and Increased Manifestation of Sex Bias in India' *Population Development Review*, 13: 77–100.

Das, D., J. Dhanoa and B. Cowan (1982), 'Exclusive Breastfeeding for Six Months: An Attainable Goal for Poor Communities', *Bulletin of the Nutrition Foundation of India*, April.

de Beauvoir, Simone (1952), *The Second Sex*, New York: Alfred A. Knop.

Devadas, R. and G. Kamalanathan (1985), 'A Woman's First Decade', paper presented at the Women's NGO Consultation for Equality, Development and Peace, New Delhi: UNICEF, April.

Engels, Friedrich (1970), 'The Origin of the Family, Private Property and the State', in K. Marx and F. Engels (eds), *Selected Works*, Vol. 3, Moscow: Progress Publishers, pp. 24–26.

Firestone, S. (1979), *The Dialectic of Sex*, London: Women's Press.

Ghosh, Shanti (1985), 'Discrimination Begins at Birth', paper presented for UNICEF Journalist's Workshop on the Female Child, New Delhi: UNICEF.

Hallberg, L. (1988), *Iron Balance in Pregnancy*, Nestle Nutrition Workshop Series 16, New York: Raven Press.

Harriss, Barbara (1986), *The Intra-family Distribution of Hunger in South Asia*, London: School of Hygiene and Tropical Medicine.

Indian Council of Medical Research (ICMR) (1982), Report of ICMR Work- ing Group, *American Journal of Clinical Nutrition*, Vol. 35, p. 1442.

International Institute for Population Sciences (IIPS) (1995), *National Family Health Survey: India, 1992–93*, Bombay.

Inkeles, Alex and David H. Smith (1974), *Becoming Modern: Individual Change in Six Developing Countries*, Cambridge: Mass Harvard University Press.

Jejeebhoy, Shireen J. (1995), *Women's Education, Autonomy, and Reproductive Behaviour: Experience from Developing Countries*, Oxford: Clarendon Press.

Jejeebhoy, Shireen J. and Saumya Rama Rao (1995), 'Unsafe Motherhood: A Review of Reproductive Health', in Monica Das Gupta, T.N. Krishnan and Lincoln C. Chen (eds), *Women's Health in India*, Delhi: Oxford University Press.

Jeffery, Patricia, Roger Jeffery and Andrew Lyon (1989), *Labour Pains and Labour Power: Women and Child Bearing in India*, New Delhi: Manohar Publications.

Khan, M.E., Richard Anker, S.K. Ghosh Dastidar and S. Bairathi (1989), 'Inequalities between Men and Women in Nutrition and Family Welfare Services: An In-Depth Enquiry in an Indian Village', in J. Caldwell and G. Santow (eds), *Selected Readings in the Cultural, Social and Behavioural Determinants of Health*, Canberra: Australian National University.

Khan, M.E. et al. (1993), 'Abortion Acceptors in India: Observations from a Prospective Study', proceedings of the International Population Conference, Montreal, International Union for Scientific Study of the Population, Belgium.

Kielmann, A.A. and Carl E. Taylor (1983), *Child and Maternal Health Services in Rural India: The Narangwal Experiment*, Vols 1 and 2, Baltimore: Johns Hopkins University Press.

Krishnaraj, Maithreyi, Ratna M. Sudarshan and Abusaleh Shariff (1999), *Gender, Population and Development*, New Delhi: Oxford University Press.

Kulkarni, Suresh N. 'Demographic and Nutritional Background of the Status of Women in India', Institute of Economic Growth, Delhi University (Mimeo Undated).

Mathur, Deepa (1985), 'Gender Dimension of Health in India', in Indu Mathur (ed.), *Health Hazards, Gender and Society*, Jaipur: Rawat Publications.

Mazumdar, Vina (ed.), *Symbols of Power: Women in a Changing Society*, New Delhi: Vikas Publications.

Miller, Barbara (1981), *The Endangered Sex: Neglect of Female Children in Rural North India*, Ithaca: Cornell University Press.

Millett, K. (1977), *Sexual Politics*, London: Virago.

Mitra, Ashok (1979), *Implications of Declining Sex Ratio in India's Population*, Bombay: Allied Publishers.

Mitra, A., L. Pathak and S. Mukherji (1980), *The Status of Women: Shifts in Occupational Participation*, New Delhi: Abhinav Publications, pp. 65–72.

Murthy, Nirmala (1982), 'Reluctant Patients: The Women of India', *World Health Forum*, Vol. 3, pp. 315–16.

Nagla, Madhu (1999), *Sociology of Medical Profession*, Jaipur: Rawat Publications.

National Institute of Population Studies (NIPS) (1992–93), *National Family Health Survey*, Bombay.

National Nutrition Monitoring Bureau (NNMB) (1980), Report for the Year 1980, Hyderabad.

National Sample Survey Organisation (NSSO) (1991), *Sarvekshana*, Vol. 15, No. 2, Department of Statistics, Ministry of Planning, Government of India, October-December.

Ortner, Sherry B. (1974), 'Is Female to Male in Nature is to Culture?' In M.Z. Rosalde and L. Lamphere (eds.) *Women, Culture and Society*, Stanford, C.A.: Standford University Press, pp. 68–67.

Padmanabha, P. (1982), 'Mortality in India: A Note on Trends and Implications', *Economic and Political Weekly*, Vol. XVII, No. 32.

Parsons, Talcott (1966), *Societies: Evolutionary and Comparative Perspectives*, Englewood Cliffs, NJ: Prentice-Hall.

Premi, M.K. (2001), 'The Missing Girl Child', *Economic and Political Weekly*, Vol. XXXVI, No. 21, 26 May.

Raman, Leela (1980), 'Amaemia in Pregnancy', in M.K. Krishna Menon, P.K. Devi and Bhaskar Rao (eds), *Postgraduate Obstetrics and Gynaecology*, Bombay: Orient Longman.

——. (1988), 'Maternal Disorders in India and their Effects on the Foetus', *Indian Journal of Paediatrics*, Vol. 47, pp. 9–17.

Rao, Saumya Rama and John W. Townsend (1999), 'Health Needs of Elderly Indian Women: An Emerging Issue', in Maithreyi Krishnaraj, Ratna M. Sudarshan and Abusaleh Shariff (eds), *Gender, Population and Development*, New Delhi: Oxford University Press.

Rogers, Barbara (1980), *The Domestication of Women: Discrimination in Developing Societies*, London: Tavistock Publications.

Sarin, A.R. (1995), 'Severe Anaemia of Pregnancy: Recent Experience', *International Journal of Gynaecology and Obstetrics*, Vol. 50, Supplement 2, October, pp. S45–49.

Sharma, S.P. and Peter Xenos (1992), 'Ageing in India: Demographic Background and Analysis based on Census Materials', Occasional Paper No. 2, Office of the Registrar General and Census Commissioner, New Delhi.

Sheshadari, S. and T. Gopaldas (1989), 'Magnitude and Implications of the Problem of Nutritional Anaemia', paper presented at the Meeting on Prevention and Control of Nutritional Anaemia, Ministry of Health and Family Welfare, New Delhi.

Shramshakti (1988), *Report of the National Commission on Self Employed Women in Informal Sector*, New Delhi: National Commission on Self Employed Women.

Srivastava, Radhika D. (2000), 'Girls are Second Class Citizens Everywhere', *The Times of India*, 17 January.

Tinker, Anne, Patricia Daly, Cynthia Green, Helen Saxenian, Rama Laxminaryanan and Kirrin Gill (1994), 'Women's Health and Nutrition: Making a Difference', World Bank Discussion Papers No. 256, Washington, DC: World Bank.

United Nations (1975), *Report of the World Conference of the International Women's Year*, Mexico City, 19 June and 2 July, p. 9.

UNICEF (1990), *Children and Women in India: A Situation Analysis*, New Delhi.

Whyte, Robert O. and Pauline Whyte (1982), *The Women of Rural Asia*, Colorado: Westview Press.

World Bank (1944), *Cataract Blindness Control Project: India*, Report No. 12246 IN, South Asia Country Department II (India), Population and Human Resources Operation Division.

——. (1996), *Improving Women's Health in India*, Washington, DC.

# 3 Gender Analysis and Population Issues

The first international conference, which was held in Bucharest (Romania) in 1974, asserted that population was a prerequisite for development. Southern countries countered that development was the best contraceptive. Ten years later, in Mexico city, the debate was nearly reversed: this time southern countries called for more family planning services to accelerate development, and the United States held that population growth was a neutral factor in economic growth. The International Conference on Population and Development, held in Cairo, Egypt in September 1994, was the arena for the most highly prepared and debated gender analysis of population issues in recent times. But, in the recent fourth World Conference on Women held in Beijing in September 1995, health became an area of concentration and debate, largely because of the consensus of Cairo conference on women's rights and health.

Women have always been the targets of population policies and programmes, because fertility is perceived as residing in women's bodies alone. Consequently, poor women, women from minority classes and castes, illiterate women, and women from labour class have all been the targets of policies aimed at reducing population growth rate in a country. In 1994, at the convening of the International Conference on Population and Development, women played a critical role in influencing the debate and were determined to do so, because so many women worldwide have been adversely affected by population policies and programmes which are primarily directed at controlling women's fertility, with little regard for women's reproductive rights or health.

According to the propagators of the international women's movement, particularly the women's health movement, and women's rights advocates, as woman has been the target for most population policies, therefore, it has been assumed as the right of the state and society to control women's bodies for achieving the desirable result in population control.

## Family Planning Programmes in India: An Assessment

India was among the earliest proponents and advocate of family planning programme. By the mid-60s, the earlier clinical approach had given rise to the motivational strategy, that is, mass education and the use of incentives and disincentives. However, the programme ends in failure, partly due to the methods then available and partly to the state's approach to the issue, female sterilization and integration of maternal and child health. This strategy never took off in the beginning because it was hospital-based and there were too few hospital deliveries. Later, because the mother and child health (MCH) component was seen only as a means to an end, it was given too little attention in terms of personnel and finance. But more importantly, even family planning services began to suffer since an element of coercion began to be associated with it. The only component of health programme specifically directed at women now became the component of programme – to limit family size.

By this time the threat of population became severe. This enabled funding agencies to widely promote family planning to the exclusion of other services, either in health or in other areas. India has by now adopted the 'cafeteria' approach with the choice of contraceptives ranging ostensibly from barrier methods such as cervical caps, etc. IUD and the pill to terminal methods. The only two methods available for men were condoms and vasectomies. Interestingly enough, the only successful method by number of acceptors was tubectomies (except during the emergency period) (Prakash, 1993). The MCH programme in the meanwhile had converted into a service distributing pills and injections – with occasional inputs of nutritional aids – for the child, and not for the mother. While the 'woman' had long been replaced by the 'mother' on the health scene, there was now a de-recognition, in practice of even the maternal role, with an emphasis on the child. Maternal mortality rates continued to be high, with the programme making hardly an impact, and the two major causes of maternal deaths were anaemia which was rooted in the general low socio-economic and cultural status of women and sepsis reflecting the failure of the medical interventions in the programme (WHO, 1991).

India's family planning programme offered a good substratum for the testing of new contraceptive methods, the most important of these being the injectable contraceptives (Baxamusa, 1985). This new method led to the women's movement worldwide. And, this was perhaps the single crucial factor in the emergence of new reproductive health strategy for the 1990s. Injectable contraceptive methods did not depend on the whims and fancies of women in order to be effective. Once they had been persuaded to accept the injection, they could not have second thoughts about it and interfere with the process. But, the injectable contraceptives also represented one more step towards taking away women's right over their bodies. But it was found that safety aspects were ignored. As problems surfaced, the women's movement which, together with a progressive and vigours health movement, had gained strength as well as acumen to challenge the medical establishment began to question the testing and promotion of the contraceptives, particularly on Third World women.

By the mid-80s it was clear that the family planning strategy was going nowhere. Reviewing the programme in 1988–89, the Public Accounts Committee's report expressed concern about the fact that although couple protection rate had gone up from 22.5 per cent in 1977 to 34.9 per cent by March 1986, the birth rate had remained stationary at 33 per cent per thousand population since 1977. Moreover, 77 per cent of the acceptors have used terminal methods with most of them having three or four children. This meant that the growing population of younger couples was not being protected and spacing methods were not being accepted (Family Welfare Programme, 1988). As an ICMR study evaluating family planning and maternal and child health services in 398 PHCs in 199 districts in India in 1987–89 showed that not only were the quality of MCH services poor, but so were the family planning services (ICMR, 1991). Yet another factor was that the maternal mortality rate had hardly registered a decrease and, worse, the largest proportion of maternal deaths was due to the anaemia which cannot be tackled at the point of pregnancy and is a reflection of the social status of women (WHO, 1991).

Among the desperate programmes of the late 80s was the Safe Motherhood Initiative, launched through the initiative of the World Bank and the WHO which continued to short-sighted the problem of motherhood and not of women. According to Prakash (1993), the three threads – the failure of the family planning programmes in the Third World, the increasing awareness of women about their health needs, mobilization of women's opinions and the articulation of their needs through the women's movement, its critique of sex-biased policy and the demand that women be participants even at the programme planning stage and the apparent recognition of what is termed women's reproductive morbidity – were woven together to evolve the reproductive health approach to women's health. It would appear that the new approach is designed to suit the long standing demands of the women's movement.

### Reproductive Health Approach

A reproductive health approach means that people have the ability to reproduce and regulate their fertility; women are able to go through pregnancy and child birth safely; the outcome of pregnancy is successful in terms of maternal and infant survival and well-being; and couples are able to have sexual relations free of the fear of pregnancy and of contracting diseases. Good reproductive health implies not only access to adequate, appropriate and good quality of reproductive health information and services, but also some knowledge of human sexuality and avoidance of high risk sexual behaviours. Reproductive health care, therefore, includes not only the treatment and prevention of diseases, but also the information and means to optimize reproductive health and family planning. The programme for action is regarded as in International Population Agreement which for the first time 'places at its center, human rights, the equality and equity of women, and reproductive health and rights' (letter from Dunlop, 1995). The gains of the Cairo conference for women are as follows:

- Recognition and a broad-based discussion internationally of the reproductive rights and reproductive health.
- Agreement on the need for the men and women to be equally responsible for reproduction and sexual behaviour, fertility and health.

- Agreement on the need to change coercive practices in family planning programmes to a broader women-centred reproductive health approach.
- Reproductive health programmes and education to include men and adolescents.
- Better delivery of reproductive health services to include full contraceptive information and choice.
- Assurance of after care and sympathetic treatment of acceptors' experiences of side effects, greater participation of women in the design, provision and management and evaluation of broader reproductive health services (Abdullah, 1994).

Reproductive health is inextricably linked to reproductive rights and freedom, and to the subject of women's status and empowerment. Thus, the reproductive health approach extends beyond the narrow confines of family planning to encompass human sexuality and reproductive health, thereby ensuring sustainable family health. In a broader context following are the issues relevant for the reproductive health approach:

### *Informed Choice and Sustainability*

Empowering both women and men to take control of their own destinies in the most intimate areas of their lives is the goal of reproductive health. There is a need to specially focus on women since they constitute the major users of reproductive health services and have the greatest problem of access, both physical and societal, to health services. Informed choice depends on woman's understanding of the options available, her intentions to carry out a particular behaviour, the extent to which she is free from controlling influences, and her ability to perform and sustain the new behaviour. A family planning client's ability to make an informed decision is enhanced when she or he understands that reproductive choice includes not only the possibility of regulating the fertility but also the option to switch contraceptive methods, discontinue use of a method or to consciously opt for pregnancy.

### *Quality of Reproductive Health Services*

Continuous concern for quality is an essential requirement for the growth of reproductive health services. Quality of reproductive health services is defined as those attributes of a service that reflect adherence to professional standards by the provider, the provision of a wide range of services in a congenial environment, and satisfaction on the part of the user. The underlying principle behind ensuring quality is to act in the interest of those who need the service. The implication of this is that improving the quality of care is a prerequisite for implementing the reproductive health approach. Individuals must be encouraged to use these services continuously rather than just initially accept them.

### *Induced Abortion and Unmet Demand*

The Medical Termination of Pregnancy (MTP) Act was passed by the Indian Parliament in 1971. However, what was thought to be a landmark in social legislation has failed to translate into reality for the majority of the Indian women, particularly in rural areas. Today, there are more illegal abortions in India than were prior to the MTP Act. This implies that there is a vast unmet need for contraception. Unsafe abortion is an important cause of maternal mortality and results in high levels of maternal morbidity in India. In large part this is due to the failure of the programme to integrate MTP services with family planning services. Women opt for non-approved centres/services for a number of reasons like apathy of doctors, poor quality of services and socio-cultural reasons, etc., therefore, effective contraception is an important means of preventing an unwanted pregnancy and pre-empting the need for abortion.

### *Women's Empowerment and Reproductive Health*

Empowering women means extending choices: choices about if and when to get married; choice about education, employment opportunities; choices about and when to get pregnant and ultimately about family size. By giving a choice and control to a woman for her own health care has a far-reaching impact on family. An essential step for improving quality of services is to give community and women's group a role in planning, implementing and monitoring reproductive health services.

### *Male Participation and Responsibility*

The participation and responsibility of the menfolk in the family planning is very essential. In many communities, female partners are unwilling or unable to seek family planning services and methods without the man's approval. The male partners are equally important in family life and they have to share fully the formation and upbringing of the children. Fathers are role models for their sons; a positive attitude can reinforce what boys are taught about responsible sexuality and respect for women.

The problem has always been that MCH programmes are not taken seriously, but are simply taken as entry points for the family planning programme. And, the very fact that the new strategy being promoted as consciously as a reproductive health strategy for women, once again, views safe motherhood as a one-point programme is indication enough of the real contents. Another dimension of the new approach is that it ignores the fact that women suffer from diseases other than that of the reproductive tract. In a study by Bang et al. (1989) women were found to have tuberculosis, suffer from malaria, iron deficiency anaemia and leprosy until then undiagnosed. A women-oriented health care strategy would acknowledge the fact that women seek help for many of these diseases much later than men do and are less likely to continue treatment.

Is there such a thing as reproductive right? Do women have to be informed that they may have a right? And if it in a culture like India, where men are presumed to have sex with their wives whenever they want and there is no concept of marital rape or forced sex, how can this concept of rights be brought into culture? Since everywhere culture has beliefs and practices about right and wrong, but in every culture the principle of beneficence is always present. Right actions are those actions that produce a balance of good consequences over bad consequences. Unsafe abortions are associated with high levels of morbidity and mortality, including infertility. By doing more harm than good, obstacles to safe abortions violate the principle of beneficence. If the woman dies or gets sick, the rest of the family is also affected. Thus, there is a need in every culture to extend the facilities of MTP services. Respect for one's culture or tradition is a good thing, except where the tradition violates human rights or fundamental ethical principles.

The Beijing conference showed that the reproductive health framework and language was more readily accepted and is the preferred language rather than reproductive rights, because conceptually it is less threatening and in practice reproductive health has much to offer given the problems of contraceptive acceptance in many population programmes. Nevertheless, implementation of the reproductive establishment is still unlikely to happen except in small measures (for example, a broadening of services some efforts at counselling and information services).

Collaboration with strong non-governmental organizations or networks with reproductive health objective would be more likely to get some success but a great deal of reorientation in family planning thinking and practices would be required. By focusing on reproductive health and addressing people's health problems, we can treat people the respect due to them as end in themselves.

Thus, this chapter attempted to provide an overview of the main elements of India's family planning programme, followed by reproductive health approach with its related issues. And, in the last it focuses on the assessment that reproductive right is one of major rights and reproductive health is one of the major perceived gains for women if serious efforts are put for their adoption.

## References

Abdullah, Rashidah (1994), 'A Women-centred Reproductive Health Model', paper presented at the International Seminar on Women's Reproductive Health, Beijing, 23–25 June, Kuala Lumpur: Asian Pacific Resource and Research Centre for Women.

Bang, R.A. et al. (1989), 'High Prevalence of Gynaecological Diseases in Rural Indian Women', *Lancet*, 14 January.

Baxamusa, Ramala M. (1984), *A Historic Perspective on Muslim Law in India, Bombay: Research Unit on Women's Studies*, Vithaldas Vidya Vihar, SNDT Women's University.

Baxamusa, Ramala (1985), 'The Price of Assistance and Kasha', Contraceptive Research in India, *SHR*, 1: 4.

Dunlop, Joan (1995), *Population and Reproductive Health: Oral History Project*, Northampton: Sophia Smith Collection (Interview).

Family Welfare Programme (1988), *139th Report of the Public Accounts Committee (1988–89)*, New Delhi: Lok Sabha Secretariat.

Indian Council of Medical Research (ICMR) (1991), *Evaluation of Quality of Family Welfare Services at Primary Health Centre Level: An ICMR Task Force Study*, New Delhi: ICMR.

Letter from Joan B. Dunlop (1995), President, International Women's Health Coalition, New York, 28 July.

Prakash, Padma (1993), 'New Approach to Women's Health Care: Means to an End?', *Economic and Political Weekly*, Vol. XXVIII, No. 51, 18 December.

World Health Organisation (WHO) (1991), *Maternal Mortality: A Global Handbook*, Geneva.

Zurayk, Huda et al. (1993), 'Concepts and Measures of Reproductive Morbidity', *Health Transition Review*, Vol. 3, No. 1.

# 4 Understanding Women's Health and Rights Issues

## A Study

The concept of right to health as a human right has recently emerged, as a result of ever growing consciousness about the dignity of human life, all over the world. Health care is considered as a socio-medical concept which implies that whatever is medically possible to promote the physical and mental well-being of the patient must be done. Medical profession, which is a noble profession, has now become a business. Medical professionals often forget their responsibilities towards their patients and conduct their professional work without observing the code of ethics and thereby violate the rights of the patients. Growing incidences of malpractices and medical negligence keep the patient at bay resulting into the poor health or sometimes in medical complications. Since women constitute nearly half of the population in any country and also have an additional responsibility of reproduction and motherhood, therefore, obviously they are more likely to be a part of a system of health care. Since health care is a socio-medical concept and not just a medical one, therefore, it does not mean mere medical treatment during illness. It means prevention, treatment and management of illness and preservation of physical and mental well-being of the person through the services provided by the medical and allied health professionals

Before any treatment or investigation, patients have the right to a clear, concise explanation in lay terms of the proposed procedure and of any available alternative procedure. Where applicable the explanation shall incorporate information on risks, side-effects or after-effects, problems relating to recuperation, likelihood of success, risk of death, and whether the proposed procedure is to be administered by or in the presence of students. A patient may refuse any treatment or investigation.

If a patient is in hospital or any other health care facility, he or she shall, unless incapacitated, be consulted about any decision to discharge or transfer to another facility. Where it is appropriate to a patient's condition or treatment, he or she shall be given advice about self-care, drug administration, special precautions which may be necessary or desirable, and the existence of special associations, facilities, aids or appliances which may be of assistance. A patient's consent shall be required before any procedure is carried out. No patient shall be treated or examined without his or her consent. However, if a patient is incapacitated and delay would be dangerous, a doctor is entitled to carry out any necessary treatment or operation. A patient's written consent shall be required for the inclusion of a patient in any research. The patient shall be adequately informed of the aims, methods, anticipated benefits and potential hazards of the study and the discomfort it may entail. The patient shall be informed that he or she is free to withdraw his or her consent to participation at any time. To ensure that the informed consent is not given under duress or from a patient in a dependent relationship to the health professional, it shall be obtained by a health professional who is not engaged in the investigation and who is completely independent of the official relationship between the patient and the health professional.

Gender disparities, which affect many women, have led to a host of health problems including unintended pregnancy, low birth weight, reproductive problems, etc. Gender consideration often leads to denial of various human rights including the access to adequate information regarding family planning and breastfeeding, informed choices for family planning sterilization, access to abortion, etc. According to the human rights conventions, which guarantee equality between sexes, many of the health disadvantages of women can be under scrutiny under equality. The present chapter, which is based on an empirical study, focuses on the understanding of women's health rights issues.

Human life is precious and every person has a fundamental right to live with dignity. It is the duty of a welfare state to protect and develop the life of every citizen and to promote his or her rights to health and medical care. Right to medical care is important because it relates to the very existence of human life. Medical care is as essential as the other basic needs of a person like food, water, shelter and clothing. Every nation has evolved its own system of laws to ensure the health rights of its citizens. These laws aim to establish a humane system of health care based on the principles of equity, justice and efficiency. By emphasizing the rights of the citizens for proper health care the welfare government tries to enhance the welfare of its people so that they can live healthy and productive lives.

Right to health and health care is also a fundamental right under Article 21 of the Constitution of India. This has also been emphasized by the Supreme Court of India in several obligations on the state to protect citizen's life from medical and other forms of negligence. However, the Consumer Protection Act, which is applicable all over India, does not fall within the category of state-level health legislation.

Reproductive health is also a matter of concern for women. There are several facets of it such as decision to conceive the child and number of children, use of different family planning methods, breastfeeding and nuances of sex-selective technology.

## Objectives

The present study is aimed to find out

- how do women adjust to possible health complications associated with abortion, family planning, sex-determination test and breastfeeding; and
- what makes them to decide for family planning and abortion and sex-determination test?

## Methodology

Interviews formed an extremely interesting and rich source of information, and made the research process a thoroughly realistic. We have tried to present the feel of the fieldwork experience by allowing the voices of some of those who were interviewed in the context of their autonomy and rights.

The following sections present the account of visits to a Family Planning Clinic in the OPD of a medical college hospital and private health facilities during our larger project of health care in May 2008. This researcher was there during clinic hours, and the women attending the clinic were being seen throughout the interview. For her, it turned out to be as much as occasion to observe as to conduct an interview. The analysis of the present study is based on some case studies gathered during the fieldwork done in relation to women with their health concerns in year 2008 in the city of Rohtak.

The chapter seeks to discuss some of these questions in the context of evidence on the understanding of women and their rights in different areas of their health concerns. It also looks into the quality of available health services, i.e., whether the women who are the acceptors are aware about other methods of contraception before the acceptance besides the awareness of possible health problems during the post-sterilization periods. Efforts have also been made to examine the follow-up visits by the health workers, and experience of post-sterilization health problems.

## Family Planning and Violation of Women's Rights

In the context of sterilization, informed consent means that the user has been aware of the other choices of methods of contraception besides the possible health problems that might occur and has been given voluntarily without any inducement, force, deceit, bias or any other form of coercion.

In view of the prevalent gender norms that rationalize the bargaining power of a woman, lack of informed choice and high infant as well as child mortality, female sterilization as a family planning measure in India raises questions about her rights.

Clients must be told that they have the option of deciding against the procedure at any time without sacrificing their right to other reproductive health services. They must also be told that a reversal of this surgery is possible, but the reversal involves a major surgery and its success cannot be guaranteed. Consent for sterilization operation should not be obtained under coercion or when the client is under physical or mental stress. It should not be obtained when a woman is sedated or when she experiences stress associated with some pregnancy-related events/problems. Clients must sign a printed application and consent form for sterilization. There are certain conditions that require doctors to be cautious, delay the surgery, refer the client to a speciality equipped centre, or counsel to opt for alternative contraception. There may be situations when it is better to counsel the female client's husband to go in for vasectomy. There are no absolute contraindications for tubectomy. Temporary contraindications include anaemia, severe hypertension, diabetes, local skin diseases, etc. The best timing for performing tubectomy is after delivery and is also called postpartum sterilization. Tubectomy can also be performed after menstrual period when pregnancy is ruled out. This procedure is called interval tubectomy. Tubectomy can also be done after the woman undergoes MTP or spontaneous abortion. Female sterilization by minilap tubectomy can be performed by a trained MBBS doctor, whereas laparoscopic sterilization can only be performed either by a gynecologist with DGO/MD/MS or a surgeon with an MS degree and trained in laparoscopy. Prior to performing a sterilization operation, a careful clinical assessment of the client should be made to ensure her fitness for surgery. Tubectomy is either done by laparotomy which entails opening of the abdomen by a small incision or by laparoscopy. Tubectomy by laparotomy is best done in the postpartum period when the operation is quite simple to perform as the uterus is large and felt per abdomen. This is a very simple and safe procedure. The operation is done at least 24 hours after delivery so that the woman has taken adequate rest and has sufficient time to make up her mind. Her haemoglobin and urine are checked pre-operatively. Consent of the woman is enough for this operation. Husband's consent is not a must for this operation. The operating doctor confirms her physical fitness for this operation before proceeding for the surgery. Tubectomy can be performed under local anaesthesia, spinal anaesthesia or general anaesthesia. Preparation for surgery includes pre-operative assessment and instructions, a review of the surgical procedure and 24-hour post-operative care. Pre-operative assessment is essential to assess the client's physical fitness for surgery and also ensures that the consent for surgery is voluntary and well informed. This assessment can also provide an opportunity for overall health screening and treatment of RTI/STDs, if required. Demographic information on age, marital status, occupation, religion, education, number of living children, sex and age of the youngest child is required to be elicited.

The women to whom we interviewed for obtaining the details regarding their entry into the hospital up to the follow-up procedures, we found that more than 70 per cent women were illiterate, therefore, they could not read the paper on which they signed before their sterilization. Nor were they informed or counselled for their sterilization in relation to the wider choices of different methods. The women are only informed that the tubectomy is the best method and, therefore, they are performing it on her for her goodness.

Before sterilization, it is mandatory for a doctor to take the history of the patient and see whether he/she is compatible for sterilization or not. However, the history which is taken is restricted only to the menstrual and obstetric history, nothing more than that. The physical examination of pelvic is also done in a causal manner without bothering for change of gloves for each patient. Urine and haemoglobin examination is also done in a routine manner. There is no cleanliness of toilets and, therefore, there are chances of infection which can be transmitted from one person to another. The operating surgeon did not conduct any final assessment of the woman before performing sterilization. There are no cases of refusal of sterilization on the basis of relative contradiction, clinical assessment or laboratory examination in the health care facility.

## Women and Sex-selection Amniocentesis Test

Amniocentesis was first introduced in India in 1974 at the All India Institute of Medical Sciences (AIIMS) in New Delhi to detect foetal abnormalities. By 1975, it was known that the test was being used for conducting sex-selective abortion. However, sex determination was banned first in 1988 in Maharashtra and then in other parts of the country. This ban, however, did not stop the lucrative business of sex-determination tests, it only made it more expensive. It was found that the violation of medical ethics by medical personnel in using technologies, which were principally meant for detecting genetic abnormalities, for detecting the sex of the foetus, and further misusing the liberal abortion laws of the country by performing sex-selective abortions (Gupta, 2000).

The amniocentesis procedure is usually performed between 14 to 20 weeks and sometimes as early as 11 weeks of pregnancy. In some cases, it may be performed in the third trimester. The third trimester risks are lower and are not linked to premature labour. Amniocentesis is also carried out to determine uterine infections in case of ruptured membranes. It also helps determine feral anaemia in babies with Rh disease. In such cases, it also helps the doctor to decide whether the foetus requires blood transfusions to save its life. During the third trimester, amniocentesis also helps assessing lung maturity. Amniocentesis is considered to be a safe procedure, but as it is an invasive diagnostic test, it has its share of risks. There are some amniocentesis risks that should be noted before carrying out the procedure. These are:

- *Miscarriage:* The rate of amniocentesis risks of miscarriage is about 1 in 300 to 1 in 500. Such risks are high if carried out before 14 weeks of pregnancy. Miscarriages happen due to infection in the uterus, the water breaks or labour is induced prematurely. Amniocentesis risks for twins or multiple pregnancy are same as the slight risk of miscarriage in normal pregnancies.
- *Cramps and vaginal bleeding:* Another risk of amniocentesis in some women is cramping and vaginal bleeding.
- *Foetal injury:* In extremely rare cases, the needle comes in contact with the baby. This may happen in case the baby moves an arm or leg and comes in contact with the needle. It is very rare to observe serious needle injuries in foetus while performing amniocentesis.
- *Rh sensitization:* Again, in rare cases, the foetal blood cells enter the mother's bloodstream triggering an immune response. This happens when the mother is Rh negative and the foetus has Rh positive blood group. The doctor may give the mother in such cases Rh immunoglobulin drugs to prevent production of antibodies against the foetal blood cells.
- *Uterine infections:* Sometimes, amniocentesis may trigger a uterine infection that may lead to miscarriage. If the mother has hepatitis B or hepatitis C, it may increase the risk of transmission to baby in first or second trimester. Amniocentesis also increases the risk of HIV from the mother being transmitted to the baby. Thus, one should avoid it in third trimester.

Another important side-effect of amniocentesis is leakage of fluid and minor irritation at the puncture site. However, the amniocentesis has some benefits too. It helps detect chromosomal abnormalities such as Trisomy 21 or Down syndrome. It also helps in detecting neural tube defects and genetic disorders. There is high level of accuracy of about 98 to 99 per cent associated with this test. The test gives the probability of birth defects, not the severity of the abnormalities. Amniocentesis also helps detect cystic fibrosis and finds whether the lungs are mature to be able to breathe on their own. Detection of DNA paternity testing before delivery, with 99 per cent accuracy rate, is also one of its major benefits.

The following reporting by a woman will make it clear that she was not informed about the health problems resulting out of the amniocentesis test:

> I had gone for the amniocentesis test in a private health clinic and found that it was a male baby, which I delivered after some time. When the child grew older, he developed a lumps in his both the hands. I consulted so many doctors, but could not get any satisfactory answer. At last, I went to AIIMS, Delhi. After taking the detail history and diagnosis of my son, they could not establish the fact that it was because of the fluid which was used at the time of performing amniocentesis test. Similar types of problems were also encountered by the other children whose mothers went for the same type of test. Now, the child has grown and is of marriageable age, and is facing a lot of problem in finding a girl. The parents of prospective girls after knowing this problem are not ready to marry them. Thus, this younger boy is facing physical as well as social problems. He often asks me, why you have done this wrong to me? However, I cogently reply that it is the technology which has done harm to you and me and made us guinea pigs for their ends.

Women go to a clinic for the test and then to another hospital for abortion. Under the MTP Act, it is difficult to prove that the woman is terminating the pregnancy merely on the ground of sex. Under the MTP Act women have the right to terminate pregnancy due to a risk to their physical and mental health, which can be caused by contraceptive failure.

> Another woman recalled her amniocentesis test experience as a nurse giving local anaesthesia and a doctor inserting a needle through the abdomen. Ultrasound monitoring during the piercing

of the amniotic sac was not followed. The doctor used a stethoscope to locate the position of foetus. They believed that the needle was inserted many times because the doctor was unable to get the fluid. During the test, the doctor had mentioned repeatedly that there were no side effects. When finished, the nurse gave them the fluid to take to a diagnostic centre for testing, which they did before going home. The woman did not know that they had faced risks of miscarriage or premature labour because amniocentesis was used without the use of ultrasound; accidental injury inflicted on the foetus by the syringe is generally responsible for such risks. She was also unaware that such procedure might have led to sepsis in the reproductive tract.

## Women and Breastfeeding

Despite being known as a breastfeeding nation, India had to enact the Infant Milk Substitute Act in 1992 to protect breastfeeding from the commercial onslaught of companies out to make a profit at the expense of the health of infants. The Act was later amended in 2003 and came to force on 1 January 2004.

The main reason that more and more mothers are turning to infant formulas is because companies selling infant food make them psychological prisoners to the belief that their product is superior to mother's milk and thus more healthy for their new born, when just the contrary is true. Any such propaganda or advertisement, allurements to doctors or medical staff is a criminal offence and punishable under the Act.

In India, very few children are breastfed one hour after birth. Though statistics suggest 96 per cent children are breastfed, only 29 per cent of the urban population and 21 per cent of the rural population are breastfed within the first hour of birth. The National Family Health Survey (NFHS)-3, published in late 2006, said that only 24.5 per cent of new mothers initiated breastfeeding in the hour after birth, 46.4 per cent breastfed exclusively the first six months and a slightly more encouraging 56.7 per cent nursed beyond six months with the introduction of complementary food. An important developmental parameter, IMR continues to stay high despite the two-decade long campaign to bring it down. Breastfeeding promotion alone contributes to 11.6 per cent reduction in IMR if coverage of promotion is 99 per cent through one-to-one and group counselling, and can avert 21.9 million disability adjusted life years at three years. With such staggering statistics lined up, the country needs to give breastfeeding an impetus. The solution is simple: promote breastfeeding by committing money and resources. If it is done more effectively, we would see more children survive, with lower rates of disease.

### *Unenforced Law and Misinformation*

If the benefits were this palpable, breastfeeding rates themselves are dismal. A study done by Breastfeeding Promotion Network of India (BPNI), headquartered in New Delhi, suggests that the main stumbling block is the lack of support for mothers from the family, society, medical fraternity and also their work places. Mothers are often asked to throw away immune-property-rich colostrums or the first milk. Older women in the family, who dictate infant feeding practices for new mothers, cite inadequate breast milk supply and encourage them to switch to infant milk substitutes. Coupled with the aggressive promotion of these substitutes through surrogate advertisements, breastfeeding rates continue to be low. Surprisingly, it is not the law that is deficient, but its implementation and formation of support structure.

The Infant Milk Substitute, Feeding Bottles and Infant Food (Regulation of Production, Supply and Distribution) Act, 1992 does not ban the products under its scope, but regulates marketing of breast milk substitutes, which the Act calls infant milk substitutes, to children under the age of two, clearly in consonance with the WHO recommendation of breastfeeding till two years.

The IMS Act aims to curtail misinformation and misdirected education of pregnant women and mothers of infants about breastfeeding, and prohibits contact between industry and pregnant women or mothers of infants. Instead of just regulating the baby food industry, the Act also mandates creating awareness among pregnant women and lactating mothers about the benefits of breastfeeding. When read with other laws like the Maternity Benefit Act, the law could adequately serve to increase breastfeeding.

Apart from benefits to the mother and child, economic value of breastfeeding is quite high. According to 1998 BPNI estimate, the value of breast milk and breastfeeding to this country of 24.4 million annual births, based on the national breastfeeding patterns over a 2-year lactation period, was around three times the national education budget then.

Using available data on lactating mothers, frequency of nursing per day in both the exclusively breastfed group and those who had introduced complementary food, the researchers indicated that Indian mothers produced an estimated total of 3,944 million litres of breast milk. If this milk were to be replaced by infant milk substitutes, it would cost $3 billion.

Little wonder then that the infant milk substitutes manufacturers have been trying to subvert the IMS Act. Surrogate advertising and sponsored medical conferences were the norm till BPNI took on food products major – Nestle – in 1994. Nestle products Cerelac and Lactogen were found to be violating provisions for advertising, labelling and sponsoring medical events. 'The Act empowers four NGOs, including BPNI, to prosecute erring companies, in addition to health officers. But, the government has done little in the way of budgetary allocation or legal support system.

In the face of a strong lobby, the government has failed to meet the targets it had set itself for the Tenth Five-Year Plan ending 2007 vis-à-vis breastfeeding (50% initiating breastfeeding, 70% exclusive breastfeeding for six months and 75 per cent complementary foods with breastfeeding till two years). And to the activists in BPNI, it is clearly the case of lack of information, of support, of skills among health workers in an institutional delivery and finally social taboos devaluing breastfeeding.

One of the women in our study reported that she was not taught the way of breastfeeding in the hospital:

> I delivered a child in the hospital. When I complained to the hospital staff for not enough milk, they did not make efforts to help for getting milk through breast. Thus, I and my child remained deprived of breastfeeding.

Another woman said:

> Since I and my baby were exposed to pain killers at birth, therefore, the feeding did not start immediately. To compensate the feeding of child, I was encouraged for the formula milk. In the mean the child and myself both felt comfortable from bottle feeding. Thus, the breastfeeding was discouraged.

Another woman reported:

> I had C-sections delivery and, therefore, the breastfeeding did not start immediately. When I returned home, I was again exposed to more taboos and misinformation and, therefore, the breastfeeding did not take place.

Breastfeeding offers health as well as emotional benefits to infants and mothers both. The baby gets protected against allergies, bonding between mother and child contributes to reduction in postpartum depression, and gives mother a rest from the reproductive cycle through lactational amenorrhoea, which has again many benefits: no anaemia, fatigue, protects against breast cancer, makes baby feel secure, and gives the baby the safest and the perfect food for full development.

### *Working Mothers and Breastfeeding*

Agriculture taking a backseat and growing urbanization has meant most of the efforts of health workers get diluted. Daily wage earners, be it agricultural labourers or construction workers, traditionally they used to take their children to work place and breastfeed on demand. Increasing contractualization of labour has meant employment practices that are not mother- and child-friendly. The woman said:

> My nutritionally breast milk go waste because I have to return to work to supplement family income. My employer forbids me to take nursing breaks or bringing my infant to the work site. Thus, I abandoned beastfeeding.

This phenomenon is equally seen in urban organized sectors. Employers – be it the state or private institutions – often do not offer a maternity leave with benefits in excess of the minimum six weeks prescribed under the Maternity Benefits Act, 1961. While the maternity leave available under this law varies from state to state with Haryana and Punjab providing for six months, others like Tamilnadu give 135 days or three months' leave. There is a long-standing demand that Act be amended to extend the minimum leave to six months and implement it uniformly in the country.

The women on whom we focused our interview reported that as and when they complained of 'not enough milk', they are usually asked to buy formula milk or stop feeding rather than making efforts for breast milk. The Infant Milk Substitutes, Feeding Bottles and Infant Foods (Regulation of Production, Supply and Distribution Act of 1992 mentions: 'Inappropriate feeding practices lead to infant malnutrition, morbidity and infant milk substitutes and related products like feeding bottles and teats do constitute a health hazard. Promotions of infant milk substitutes and related products have been more extensive and pervasive than the dissemination of information concerning the advantages of mother's milk and breastfeeding and contributes to decline in breastfeeding'.

Breastfeeding and its success depends on hormonal control, particularly the flow of the mother's milk, which depends on her state of mind. If there is any doubt planted in her mind about her ability to lactate, it is unlikely that she will succeed. Therefore, health workers or care providers have to play a vital role in building up the confidence of new mothers. However, such support is rarely forthcoming. If a woman complains of 'not enough milk' she is usually asked to buy a formula feed rather than helped to gain confidence (Gupta, 2008).

## Women and Abortion

### *Medical Termination of Pregnancy Act*

Abortion has been made legal in India since 1972, when the Medical Termination of Pregnancy Act was passed. Under the Act, abortion is legal if it involves a risk to the life of the woman or causes grave injury to her physical or mental health or is likely to result in the birth of a baby with physical or mental abnormalities or is a result of rape or contraceptive failure. The Act further states that abortions could take place in government approved health facilities specifically approved for conducting such abortions and by registered medical practitioner.

Data providing consistent estimates of induced abortions in India are scarce: whatever is available is through government reports and surveys. Available abortion statistics shows that five to six million abortions occur every year in unapproved facilities (Ganatra, 2000; Arnold et al., 2002). Illegal abortions are eight to eleven times as high as legal abortions (Chhabra, 1996; Jessani and Iyer, 1995; Chhabra and Nuna, 1994).

In the Medical Termination of Pregnancy Act, it is the medical doctor who decides whether or not an abortion seeker fulfils the criteria spelled out in the Act. It is again the doctor who decides as to how liberally or restrictively to interpret the Act in a given socio-political context. In addition to other factors, service provider's attitude towards and understanding of women and their abortion needs influence the interpretation of the Act and is an important variable influencing women's access to abortion services. Bandewar (2003) finds that the pattern of abortion practice indicates that perceptions and concerns for women's health in the context of their abortion needs do not go with their abortion care service pattern. This is because a large number of service providers have mentioned that it was not advisable for women to use abortion as spacing method. One expects that they would provide contraceptive counselling to women seeking abortion care to avoid repeat abortions. Contraceptives were forced without leaving much space for making informed choices and denying opportunities to educate themselves vis-à-vis contraceptives.

However, the gap between perceptions and practices could be better explained with the help of forces at work which are pushing medical care service sector towards its commodification. Commercial interests of the medical community in abortion service provision in particular can further explain these gaps. Combating the irrational and unethical abortion care practices in isolation without understanding the dynamics of the larger health care system will be a difficult and perhaps even futile task. Further, this is complemented by the convenient patriarchal attitudes towards women-specific health care needs, such as abortion care needs. One of the women reports:

> When I became pregnant for third time I decided to go for abortion. I with a neighbour went to civil hospital. The lady doctor agreed for abortion but said that you must accept sterilization also. I became very much nervous. I did not want to go through operation and hence came back.

One woman said that doctors have a different opinion about the legality of the abortion:

> One of the doctors said that just because abortion is legalized, it does not mean that they should be so liberal in doing this.

### *Unsafe Abortions*

The Mumbai High Court judgment disallowing the abortion of a 26-week-old foetus has sparked off a nationwide debate on abortion and a woman's right of choice. But, for a majority of Indian women, medical termination of pregnancy (MTP, the medical term for abortions) remains largely unsafe.

Unsafe abortions are those that performed illegally, by untrained practitioners with faulty equipment, leading to injuries, infections and even death. India has the highest number of unsafe abortions in the world. According to National Rural Health Mission (NRHM) estimates, abortion-related deaths contribute to 8 per cent (approximately 4,600 deaths annually) of all maternal deaths in India. The irony is apparent when doctors say MTP, if done right, is among the safest medical procedures. Of the 6.4 million abortions performed in India in 2002 and 2003, 56 per cent or 3.6 million were unsafe, says the Abortion Assessment Project I, 2004. The study – one of the largest in recent times – was managed by the Mumbai-based Centre for Equity into Health and Allied Themes and Health Watch Trust. It included qualitative and quantitative studies conducted across various states by non-governmental organizations (NGOs), researchers and health care professionals.

It also pointed out problems of reach and access with public investment in abortion facilities being woefully inadequate. Only 25 per cent of abortion facilities in the organized sector are government-owned; the rest are private clinics. These are so expensive that they completely exclude the poor sections.

'There's inadequate, inequitable distribution of facilities for safe abortions. Contraceptive usage is low in India, hence the great demand for safe abortion services,' said Dr Jaydeep Tank, chairperson of the MTP Committee at the Federation of Obstetric and Gynaecological Societies of India (FOGSI). Besides, only 6 per cent of India's 23,000 primary health centres (PHCs) provide abortion services. 'Besides risk to life, unsafe abortions have serious long-term repercussions like life-long disabilities and reproductive tract infections,' said Sushanta Banerjee, senior advisor at Ipas, an NGO.

For a country with a 'liberal' law on abortion, Banerjee further said that awareness about it is extremely low even three decades after it was enacted. 'In Jharkhand, for instance, we found that 82 per cent of women didn't even know that abortion was legal,' he said. In a related study by the Population Council in Rajasthan in 2002, the figure was 84 per cent and in Maharashtra at least 37 per cent of those who had had abortions thought they were illegal. This misconception leads many women to unqualified professionals. Other barriers to safe abortion are 'social stigma and myths attached to MTP', said Tank. 'Awareness about abortion through drugs like Mifepristone and Misoprostol is also low, despite they being legal and easily available.'

Social barriers like spousal consent and judgmental doctors are also deterrents, though the law requires no such consent. Under the government's Reproductive and Child Health Project, safe abortions are a key concern and some progress is being made – maternal mortality due to abortion was 11 per cent in 2001. 'We need to generate awareness at the community level about contraception and safe abortion, in both rural areas and urban slums,' said Thomas Chandy, CEO, Save the Children in India. Ipas also advocates training of mid-level service providers like nurses and non-allopathic doctors in remote areas where access to trained doctors is a problem.

Only two in five of the estimated 6.4 million abortions that take place annually in India are safe. The number of women aborting an unwanted child has dipped globally. But, the rate of unsafe terminations continues to be almost as bad. Around 41.6 million women underwent abortions in 2003 compared to 45.5 million in 1995 – a drop to 29 per 1,000 women from 35 (*The Times of India*, 14 October 2009).

Abortion remains highly restricted, and unsafe abortion is common and continues to damage women's health. The evidence is strong that empowering women with the means to decide for themselves when to become pregnant and how many children to have significantly lowers unintended pregnancy rates and thereby reduces the need for abortion.

Medical termination of pregnancy is a legal provision provided to women. Liberalization of abortion has led to the fact that women are all aware that they can get an MTP done literally on demand any time.

In one study, Das, Rai and Singh (2004) found that medical termination of pregnancy was done also with laparoscopic legations, in contravention to medical standards. A bicycle pump with a nasal tube attached to its end was used to pump air into the abdomen, and in some cases, the bulb of a blood pressure instrument was used to pump air. Carbon-dioxide was not used at all.

## Conclusion

The chapter falls in three main parts. The first part reflects on the understanding of women's health rights, the second in the context of different parameters of woman's health where she is directly relating herself to health, i.e., women and family planning; women and breastfeeding; women and abortion; and women and sex-selection test. Finally, the paper concludes by problematizing the autonomy and right of the women in the above context.

The women need urgent attention in the broader context of individual freedom and human ethics. Data from the District Level Household Survey-Reproductive and Child Health (2002–04) covering a nationally representative sample of 5,07,622 currently married women aged 15–44 years, has been used for the present analysis. Bivariate and multivariate analyses have been performed to identify the factors associated with female sterilization acceptance within the broader framework of ethical issues. Although about one-third of Indian women use sterilization as a method for regulating fertility, analysis reveals that people from different socio-economic, religious and demographic strata do not generally opt for sterilization in equal proportion. Informed choice has found to be very poor among women and so also the quality of available services. The need of the hour is to offer choices and quality services. Besides sensitizing the providers about the importance of ethical issues, the government must think over improving information education and communication, better quality services, and importance on spacing methods.

## References

Arnold, F. et al. (2002), 'Sex-Selective Abortions in India', *Population and Development Review*, Vol. 28, No. 4, pp. 759–85.

Balagopal, Gayathri (2009), 'Access to Health Care among Poor Elderly Women in India: How Far Do Policies Respond to Women's Realities?', *Gender and Development*, Vol. 17, Issue 3, pp. 481–91.

Bandewar, Sunita (2003), 'Abortion Services and Providers' Perceptions: Gender Dimensions', *Economic and Political Weekly*, Vol. XXXVIII, No. 21, p. 2081.

Beser, E., V. Aydemir and H. Boxkaya (1994), 'Body Mass Index and Natural Age at Menopause', *Gynecologic and Obstetric Investigation*, Vol. 37, No. 1, pp. 40–42.

Bhatt, Rohit V. (1991), 'Camp Laparoscopic Sterilization Deaths in Gujarat State, India, 1978–1980', *Asia-Oceania Journal of Obstetric and Gynaecology*, Vol. 17, No. 4, pp. 297–301.

Brambilla, D.J. and S.M. McKinlay (1989), 'A Prospective Study of Factors Affecting Age at Menopause', *Journal of Clinical Epidemiology*, Vol. 42, pp. 1031–39.

Bromberger, I.T., K.A. Mathews and L.H. Kuller (1997), 'Prospective Study of the Determinants of Age at Menopause', *American Journal of Epidemiology*, Vol. 145, pp. 124–33.

Chhabra, R. (1996), 'Abortion in India: An Overview', *Demography India*, Vol. 25, No. 1, pp. 83–92.

Chhabra, R. and S.C. Nuna (1994), *Abortion in India: An Overview*, New Delhi: Ford Foundation.

Das, Abhijit, Ramkant Rai and Dinesh Singh (2004) 'Medical Negligence and Rights Violation', *Economic and Political Weekly*, Vol. XXXIX, August 28–September 3.

Ellen, B.G., J. Bromberger, S. Crawford, S. Samuels, G.A. Greenndale, S.D. Harlow and J. Skurnick (2001), 'Factors Associated with Age at Natural Menopause in a Multi-ethnic Sample of Middle Women', *American Journal of Epidemiology*, Vol. 153, No. 9, pp. 856–74.

Ganatra, B.R. (2000), 'Abortion Research in India: What We Know, and What We Need to Know', in Radhika Ramasubban and Shireen J. Jejeebhoy (eds), *Women's Reproductive Health in India*, Jaipur: Rawat Publications.

Gupta, Arun (2008), 'Manipulation by Assistance: Undermining Breastfeeding', *Economic and Political Weekly*, Vol. XLIII, No. 36, 6 September, p. 12.

Gupta, Jyotsna Agnihotri (2000), *New Reproductive Technologies: Women's Health and Autonomy*, New Delhi: Sage Publications.

Jacob, K.S. (2009), 'Caste and Inequalities in Health', *The Hindu*, 22 August.

Jessani, A. and A. Iyer (1995), 'Abortions: Who is Responsible for Her Rights?', in Malini Karkal (ed.), *Our Lives, Our Health*, Coordination Unit, New Delhi, The World Conference on Women, Beijing.

Luoto, R., J. Kaprio and A. Uutela (1994), 'Age at Natural Menopause and Socio-demographic Status in Finland', *American Journal of Epidemiology*, Vol. 139, pp. 64–76.

Mane, Purnima (2008), 'Population, Gender Inequality and Health: India in a Global Context', *Demography India*, Vol. 37, No. 2, p. 176.

National Sample Survey Organisation (1998), Maternal and Child Health Care in India, 52nd Round.

Pandey, Arvind (2008), 'Population, Gender and Health', *Demography India*, Vol. 37, No. 2, pp. 167–69.

Papanek, V. (1984), *Design for the Real World: Human Ecology and Social Change*, London: Thames and Hudson.

Patel, Vibhuti (1992), 'Review of the Effects of the Structural Adjustment Programme on Women', Unpublished paper presented to the Development Studies Institute, London School of Economics, 27 November.

Rosenzweig, Mark R. and T. Paul Schultz (1982), 'Market Opportunities, Genetic Endowments, and Intra-family Resource Distribution: Child Survival in Rural India', *The American Economic Review*, Vol. 72, No. 4, pp. 803–15.

Shah, Rashmi S. (1998), 'Menopause ad HRT: Growing Public Health Challenges', *ICMR Bulletin*, Vol. 28, No. 1, January.

Standford, J.L., P. Harge and L.A. Brinton (1987), 'Factors Influencing the Age at Natural Menopause', *Journal of Chronic Diseases*, Vol. 40, pp. 995–1002.

Syamala, S. and M. Sivakami (2005), 'Menopause: An Emerging Issue in India', *Economic and Political Weekly*, Vol. XL, No. 47, 19–25 November.

*The Times of India* (2009), 14 October.

World Bank (2002), *World Development Indicators 2002*, Washington, DC.

Wyon, John Benjamin and John Everett Gordon (1971), *The Khanna Study: Population Problems in the Rural Punjab*, Cambridge: Harvard University Press.

# 5 Women and Health Issues under Law

As stated in the previous chapter, human life is precious and every person has a fundamental right to live with dignity. It is the duty of a welfare state to protect and develop the life of every citizen and to promote his or her rights to health and medical care. Right to medical care is important because it relates to the very existence of human life. Medical care is as essential as the other basic needs of a person like food, water, shelter and clothing. Every nation has evolved its own system of laws to ensure the health rights of its citizens. These laws aim to establish a humane system of health care based on the principles of equity, justice and efficiency.

Right to health and health care is a fundamental right under Article 21 of the Constitution of India. This has also been emphasized by the Supreme Court of India in several of its rulings. Article 21 of the Constitution casts a special obligation on the state to protect citizen's life from medical and other forms of negligence.

The Fourth World Conference on Women stated that women have the right to the enjoyment of the highest attainable standard of physical and mental health. The enjoyment of this right is vital to their life and well-being and their ability to participate in all areas of public and private life. Health has been defined by WHO as a state of complete physical, mental and social well-being and not merely the absence of disease or infirmity (WHO, 1946). Thus, women's health should also involve their emotional, social and physical well-being and is determined by the social, political and economic context of their lives, as well as biology. Prevailing laws ensure the well-being of women and grant them equal status in the society.

When we discuss laws related to women's health, it needs to be emphasized that we have to deal with health in its comprehensive meaning. Thus, not only laws specifically related to women's physical, mental or social health are important, but even the laws that empower women are also relevant. This is because women's empowerment is an undisputed determinant of women's health.

Article 42 of the Constitution of India provides: 'The State shall make provision for securing just and humane conditions of work and for maternity relief'. And further: 'The State shall regard the raising of the level of nutrition and the standard of living of its people and the improvement of health as among its primary duties and in particular. The State shall endeavour to bring about prohibition of the consumption except for medicinal purposes of intoxicating drinks and of drugs which are injurious to health' (Article 47).

With few exceptions, most laws in India make no distinction between male and female in the area of health. This paper proposes to focus on certain laws related to women's health issues and some other emerging areas which still do not have legislation but are already under the moral and ethical debate. The protectionist kind of laws would include Maternity Benefit Act, Medical Termination of Pregnancy Act, and Pre-Natal Diagnostic Termination Act. Issues related to family planning methods and reproductive technology will also be dealt.

## Maternity Benefit Act, 1961

As the number of women employers is increasing, this piece of legislation was passed with the object of doing social justice to women workers employed in factories, mines and plantations. It is basically meant to provide maternity leave and other benefits to women employees and enabling them to fulfil their commitment to nursing their babies till attainment of an age of 15 months.

The Act prohibits the employer from engaging or making a woman work for six weeks after her delivery or miscarriage. The employer is also required not to engage a woman in an arduous task, one which involves hours of standing on or which in any way is likely to interfere with her pregnancy, the normal development of the foetus or is likely to cause miscarriage or otherwise adversely affect her health provided she requests the employer to this effect. This stipulation applies to one month before the date of her expected delivery, or any six weeks before the expected delivery. Woman has a right to payment of maternity benefit for the three months. To claim this benefit of wages, however, she must have been in employment for at least eighty days in the twelve months immediately preceding the date of their expected delivery. A woman is also entitled to medical bonus of ₹ 250 if no pre-natal confinement and post-natal care is provided free of charge by the employer. This applies also to a woman who has miscarriage. A woman is also entitled to leave for a month for any illness arising out of the pregnancy, delivery, premature delivery or miscarriage. The medical bonus may be revised from time to time in keeping with the cost of living.

In case of miscarriage or MTP, a woman is entitled to six weeks' leave with pay at the rate of maternity benefit immediately following the day of her miscarriage/MTP on production of proof thereof. Section 9A provides for leave with wages for a period of two weeks immediately following tubectomy. A woman suffering from illness arising out of pregnancy, delivery, premature birth of child, miscarriage, MTP, tubectomy operation and the like is entitled to one month's additional leave with wages at the rate of maternity benefit of her entitlements under Sections 6 and 9.

The Act also stipulates that she is allowed two nursing breaks in the course of her work till the child attains fifteen months independent of the normal breaks.

A woman cannot be dismissed during the period of her pregnancy nor can any retrograde steps be initiated with regard to the terms and conditions of service. The only exception being on account of gross misconduct where the employer may, by an order in writing communicated to the women, deprive her maternity benefit and/or medical bonus. The woman, however, has the right to appeal to the prescribed authority within a period of 60 days. The employer cannot deduct the wages of a woman entitled to maternity benefit because of the nature of work assigned to her by virtue of the provisions contained in Section 4(3) or for breaks allowed for nursing the child under Section 11.

The Act is applicable to factories, mines and plantations. The government can also by notification extend its applicability to other classes of establishment – industrial, commercial, agricultural or otherwise.

The Government of India has recently increased the maternity leave entitlement from 90 days to 135 days. Fifteen days' paternity leave to fathers has also been provided for.

Strangely, the statute provides for forfeiture of maternity benefit. If a woman works in the establishment during the period of authorized absence, her claim to maternity benefit can be forfeited. In the prevailing unequal situation some employers force their employees to work and take refuge under this provision. The Act provides for inspectors empowered to examine its violation. A few years ago, a circular was issued to Central Government employees restricting the benefits to married women. This caused various protests and the circular was withdrawn. Such a move was clearly against the spirit of the Act which recognizes the women's right to health and does not concern itself with existing norms of morality and is truly a welfare legislation (Ramaseshan, 1999). The Act also mentions about the provision of crèches for children at working place. But the highest body of country, i.e., the parliament still does not have any provision of crèche. The Act also provides a clean work environment, effective ventilation and temperature, and all other amenities. Conversely, in most of the establishments, the laws are blatantly violated.

## Pre-Natal Diagnostic Techniques (Regulation and Prevention of Misuse) Act, 1994

This Act provides for regulation of the pre-natal diagnostic techniques for the purpose of detecting any genetic or metabolic disorder, chromosomal abnormalities or certain congenital malformations and sex-linked disorders and prevention of misuse of such techniques for the purpose of pre-natal sex determination for female foeticide. The Act thus aims at preventing the killing of baby girls even before they are born. However, it is doubtful whether the practice of pre-natal sex determination followed by abortion in case of female child has decreased to any significant extent.

Maharashtra was the first state to pass the Pre-Natal Diagnostic Techniques (PNDT) Act in 1988 under public pressure.

The Act bans the use of medical techniques and technologies for pre-natal diagnostics except in cases where the pregnant woman is above 35 years of age, has a history of two or more abortions or foetal loss, has a history of being exposed to potentially teratogenic drugs, radiation, infection or hazardous chemicals or has a family history of mental retardation or physical deformities. The Act also declares illegal any advertisement regarding the availability of pre-natal sex detection facilities at clinics, laboratories or centres. The regulation of these centres is to be achieved through bodies appointed by government.

Informed consent of the pregnant woman has to be taken and also a copy of the same to be given to her before such tests can be conducted. The Act also prohibits disclosure of the sex of the foetus to the woman or her relatives by words, signs or any other manner.

The Act defines offences and lays down penalties for contravention of its provisions. A significant aspect is that under Section 24, unless the contrary is proved, the court shall presume that the pregnant woman has been compelled by her husband or the concerned relative to undergo pre-natal diagnostic tests and such person shall be liable for punishment for abetment of the offence. The Act makes an offence under the Act cognizable, non-bailable and non-compoundable.

The country has seen its first ever conviction for foetal sex determination after 12 years of existence of PNDT Act, first time in Haryana, when a doctor and his assistant have been given two years imprisonment and a fine of ₹ 5,000 each for violating the PNDT Act, 1994 (*Tribune*, 28 March 2006). Another such conviction was in Punjab for improper maintenance of records and the doctor got away with a fine. According to Sabu George (2006), 'Sex selection is a high volume, low risk business. Volumes have to be high because one or two cases do not get the errant doctor much money and the risk low because hardly anyone is caught.' According to Dr Bedi (2006), 'It is a ₹ 500–1,000 crore industry if you take into account that five to seven lakh foetuses are aborted in the country every year at a cost of ₹ 10,000–15,000 each. So doctors won't stop conducting ultrasound tests till there is deterrent.' The deterrent will also come in the form of the convicted doctor losing his/her registration. Debarring is inherent in the law.

## Medical Termination of Pregnancy Act, 1971

The issue of reproduction has always been central to a woman's life. In all cultures and ages women have sought ways and means to either prevent conception, or get rid of an unwanted pregnancy, or to voluntarily remain child free, or to deal with involuntary childlessness. Intervention in reproduction is not of recent origin. Contraception and abortion have been known for long time. Up until the Middle Ages in Europe (and in developing countries to some extent even until this day), women practised as healers and midwives, providing contraceptive measures, performing abortions and offering concoctions to ease the pain of labour, according to methods and skills handed down from generation to generation.

An extremely significant development took place with the passing of the Medical Termination of Pregnancy (MTP) Act in 1971 which became effective from April 1972. Until then, the abortion laws in India had been very restrictive. The most important reason given for liberalization was to counter the hazard of the large number of illegal abortions. Since the concept of family planning was already accepted, it was assumed that the liberalization of the abortion law would meet with support rather than opposition from religious and professional groups. The legislation provided recourse to abortion under broad health (physical and mental) grounds on eugenic indications, under juridical conditions (such as incest or rape), and for social reasons such as mental or social injury to the mother. The law did not have population control as its stated objective. However, the provisions of the law were liberal enough for those who wished to avail themselves of it to do so. The committee to study the question of abortion legislation, appointed by Ministry of Health and Family Planning, Government of India (1966) stated: '… abortion also can be used as a means to control family size as is being done currently in several countries, in which family planning or contraception and abortion are in two parallel categories, both of which lead to population control.' It is noteworthy that Indian women obtained the right to abortion without a struggle or even a campaign on this issue, whereas it is still an explosive issue in many countries, predominantly Catholic countries as well as in the US where the opposition to abortion is the strongest and is organized in a pro-life lobby. The population control motive is likely to have played an important role in the liberalization of abortion in India. The easy availability of abortion did not make it an issue of 'self-determination' for women in India (Gupta, 2000).

During the past three decades, there has been liberalization of abortion laws throughout the world. In India, abortions were governed exclusively by the Indian Penal Code and the Code of Criminal Procedure. It was considered a crime except when performed to save the life of a pregnant woman.

The MTP Act is a health care measure which helps to reduce maternal morbidity and mortality resulting from illegal abortions. It also affords an opportunity for motivating such women to adopt some form of contraception. It was enacted purely to safeguard the rights of women and the doctors who performed abortion. Previously, abortion was an offence under the Indian Penal Code except when it was done to save the life of woman. This led to illegal abortions. According to the objects and reasons of the Act, doctors had often been confronted with gravely ill or pregnant women whose uterus has been tempered with a view to causing an abortion who consequently suffered very severely. The legislation was conceived (1) as a health measure – where there is danger to life or risk to physical or mental health of the woman, (2) on humanitarian grounds such as when a lunatic woman was raped, etc., and (3) eugenic grounds where there is a substantial risk that the offspring would suffer from deformities and diseases.

The MTP Act allows abortion if the doctor is of opinion that the continuance of the pregnancy would endanger the life of the pregnant woman or involve grave injury to her physical or mental health, or there is a substantial risk that the child would suffer from disabling physical or mental abnormalities. The anguish caused by pregnancy as a result of rape, or of failure of any device limiting the number of children may be presumed to constitute a grave injury to the woman's mental health. The medical practitioner can take into account the pregnant woman's actual or reasonable foreseeable environment to determine the advisability of abortion. If the pregnancy is 12 weeks old, the opinion of one registered medical practitioner is sufficient but for pregnancy of between 12 and 24 weeks, the opinion of two registered medical practitioners is required. In theory the law recognizes women's right to abortion, as the medical practitioner has to consider only her consent. The matter is thus purely between the two and even the husband's consent becomes unnecessary. In reality, however, a woman's right to abortion is very restricted, and mostly, it turns out to be a family decision. Various court judgments have hold that abortion of a foetus without the husband's consent would amount to cruelty under the Hindu Marriage Act and hence is a ground for divorce.

Under the MTP Act, the pregnancy of a girl below 18 years or that of a lunatic can be terminated only with the consent in writing of her guardian. The Act permits the pregnancy of a 'lunatic' (as defined under the Lunacy Act and hence will include the mentally ill and mentally disabled) with the written consent of her guardian provided the doctor is of the opinion that the pregnancy will cause injury to the woman's physical or mental health. No law permits sterilization to be performed on the mentally ill or disabled. The issue is complex, involving a woman's right over her body. Besides, given over utter callousness towards the underprivileged, any such freedom to perform sterilization will be misused. Besides, there are degrees of retardation and some women are capable of taking care of themselves through in a limited way. At the same time, there is genuine anguish of many parents that their mentally retarded daughters might become victims of pregnancy due to sexual abuse and about their daughter's hygiene after their lifetime.

The MTP Act also recognizes 'failure of contraceptives' as a ground for seeking abortion. This relief is restricted, however, to married women. Unwed pregnant women are forced to mention rape or grave injury to mental or physical health in order to seek abortion. Since the rules in government hospitals are rigid, such women prefer to go to private clinics or quacks.

In India, merely the fact that abortion legislation is liberal does not guarantee that women have access to legal abortion facilities. Incidence of illegal abortions is alarmingly high. It is ten times as many as illegal abortions are carried out as legal ones and at least 80 per cent of women admitted to hospital with complications have had abortions performed by unqualified people. Around one-tenth of maternal deaths in the country are due to septic abortions. About seven million induced abortions take place every year. Abortion is advocated openly by government authorities (Nair, 1991). One hoarding spotted in Bombay read: 'Carrying again? You need not worry. Get your pregnancy terminated. Abortion is legal'. It is clear that abortion is regarded by the authorities as a family planning method. On paper, however, abortion is not part of the family planning programme and is ostensibly only a health measure (Nair, 1991). Studies show that high percentage of women seeks help for abortion at a late stage of pregnancy (Grand, 1992). This is due to reasons of their legal rights to abortion, ignorance regarding the availability of legal abortion facilities and above all due to inadequate health care facilities and above all due to inadequate health care services (Toubia, 1991: 12; quoted in Hunt, 1992: 4). Mainly the better educated/informed and economically well-off women find their way to legal abortion clinics, while women who are either less educated and/or economically weak fall back on illegal abortion services, providers of which also have a generally low educational level and many not themselves understand the instructions for correct use of the abortion pill. These women could use it without the supervision of trained health workers. They are less likely to have access to the necessary information. When complications occur, medical help will often be inaccessible to them (Grand, 1990).

Although induced abortion was legalized in India in 1971, the number of legal abortions in India has risen rapidly since 1972, and it has levelled off at about 6,00,000 annually (MoHFW, 1992). The fact that many legal abortions performed in private facilities are probably not reported may affect the data. In addition, a number of illegal abortion procedures are in use – from modern surgical techniques carried out by private practitioners without the requisite licences to a variety of folk methods. The actual numbers of illegal, unsafe abortions performed and the extent of associated morbidity and mortality are unknown. In one hospital study infection resulting from abortion was the single highest cause of death (26% of direct obstetric deaths and 18% of deaths from all causes) (Rao, 1988). In community-based studies of Andhra Pradesh and Karnataka, illegal abolitions were estimated to be responsible for about 6 and 3 per cent of total maternal deaths, respectively (Reddy, 1992; Bhatia, 1988). The studies indicated that about two-thirds of all abortion deaths involved induced abortions and the other third miscarriages. According to the Andhra Pradesh study, roughly half of the abortion deaths were caused by haemorrhage and the other half by infection. The Indian Council of Medical Research (1988) carried out a study of induced abortions in the states of Haryana, Orissa, Rajasthan, Tamil Nadu and Uttar

Pradesh in 1983–84 and found that for the five states combined, 6 of each 1,000 pregnancies ended in legal abortions whereas 213 in illegal abortions. Assuming this relationship holds for subsequent years for the rest of India, the approximately 6,00,000 legal abortions reported in 1990 indicate that a total of about 1.3 million illegal abortions are performed annually in the country. For the five states combined, only about 55 per cent of the abortions were carried out in the first trimester, and of these only about one-quarter were provided by doctors (government or private) or other health staff. A study funded by the Ford Foundation argues that previous research seriously underestimates the magnitude of illegal abortions and suggests that nearly 7 million induced abortions occur annually. These figures imply that for every legal abortion in India, 10 more are performed illegally. The study also estimates that the number of abortion-related deaths is significantly higher than was previously reported, accounting for at least 15 per cent of all maternal deaths (Chhabra and Nuna, 1994). Thus, it is clear that medical terminations performed by qualified personnel, which are often performed at facilities distant from women's homes and may be prohibitively expensive, are competing with more convenient, less expensive alternatives performed locally, which many believe are less dangerous for women than surgical techniques. The constraints involved in delivering medical terminations suggest that increasing the number of procedures performed at public sector facilities will require an increase in the number of approved facilities, improvements in the quality of services provided, and public education. Devolving authority from specialists and training a wider range of health providers to perform terminations in the first trimester can also make these services more available, to spare women the complications and deaths associated with unsafe practices, particularly in rural areas. The complications of unsafe abolitions should be promptly referred and treated. The high levels of abortion in India underscore the need to make contraceptives more widely available so that women can avoid unwanted pregnancies in the first place (World Bank, 1996).

## Family Planning Methods

The use of condom to prevent conception has been known for a long time. Besides, abstinence, withdrawal and other traditional practices also contributed to birth control. Research in animal and human reproduction made great strides in the 20th century. With the development of the contraceptive pill in the early 1990s, and later, other contraceptive methods, fertility management through medical technology became more efficient and reliable.

According to guidelines of the Helsinki Declaration, in any research on human beings, each potential subject must be adequately informed of the aims, methods, anticipated benefits and potential hazards and the discomfort if any. This is to prevent human beings from becoming guinea pigs. Various methods of family planning like pills, injectable contraceptives, implants and sterilization will be discussed below for the purpose of women's health issues.

### *Pills*

The one area where there is a need to examine a legislation is in the field of family planning. The pill, which has been in the market since the 1960s, was considered safe for long, as its side effects came to be known much later. Unlike in the West where it is not available without a doctor's prescription, in India, pills like Mala-D are available over the counter and marketed with an aggressive advertising campaign by the government-sponsored media. While this will be no doubt beneficial to women as they would be examined on an individual basis, in reality medical facilities are unavailable or difficult to reach for a large number of women. In such a case a rigid rule might make even the existing facilities inaccessible to the average woman who does not want a pregnancy.

### *The Injectable Contraceptives*

One of the injectables is Net-en and its import has been permitted since late 1984. Net-en is a bimonthly injection that inhibits the production of gonadotropin. It does not need any chart as in the case of pill or periodic check-ups as in IUDs. In March 1985, research trials of Net-en were to be held at a Rural Health Centre in Patancheru, the *Stree Shakti Sangathana* tried to dissuade the doctors from conducting trail as they had read about the side effects of the drugs and the lack of adequate long-term studies with it. They found that the women recruited for the trial were only told that they would not conceive if they took the drug, but were not told about its side effects nor that they were participating in a trial (Balasubrahmanyan, 1986). The case is still in the court.

Depo Provera is another injectable contraceptive that is available without a prescription. Both these drugs are the subject matter of litigation. In the absence of any legislation to define and regulate such contraceptives (many of them prohibited in the countries of their origin or sold under strict conditions) activist groups have been forced to take these issues to court. Depo Provera has now been approved for use. Earlier it was not approved for use in India on the grounds that its use as a contraceptive was banned in the country of its origin (Prakash, 1986; Balasubrahmanyan, 1986). The government gave its approval in 1994 and launched in India.

Women's health advocates have expressed their concern over unethical manner in which trials have been conducted. They point out the unsuitability of introducing hormonal injectable contraceptives in mass programme, where it is difficult to follow up users for adverse effects and provide relief. They also doubt the objectivity of post-marketing studies of a drug due to the interests that stand to profit from its extensive use. They have pointed out the risks involved in introducing injectable contraceptives in the context of family planning programme (Balasubrahmanyan, 1986). There are number of contradictions for the use of these drugs, but primary health centres in India have hardly any facilities for such large-scale investigation and maintenance of records. Moreover, the staff is often poorly-trained callous or careless, and under compulsion to meet impossible targets, which creates a great potential for abuse. There is an absence of hygienic conditions, including clean needles and syringes and a lack of follow-up facilities.

### *Implants*

Work on contraceptives in the form of implants first began in the 1960s. The idea was to find a way to put hormones in some kind of capsule that would gradually release them into the body over a period of time to prevent pregnancy. A number of different hormones and different types of capsules were tested, as well as different sites on the body for places to implant. The most widely used is Norplant. Norplant has been tested and used mainly in less developed countries.

Contraindications for Norplant use as listed in the manual for clinicians by the Population Council (1990) include cardiovascular disorders, abnormal vaginal bleeding without a known cause, benign or malignant tumours, and known or suspected breast cancer. Among the most frequently reported side effects are changes in menstrual bleeding. About 60 per cent of Norplant users suffer disruption of their menstrual cycles, including prolonged bleeding, spotting and amenorrhea. Other so-called 'minor' side effects include severe headaches, nausea, dizziness, weight gain or loss, nervousness and depression, scarring, acne and other skin disorders and infections at the implantation site (Nair, 1991).

Norplant pre-introduction studies were held in 1984 but abandoned after two years but once again in 1993, fresh trials of Norplant (R) started in ten medical colleges all over India under the auspices of the ICMR. These trials are being funded by various international organizations, including USAID and the IPPF. The results of the earlier Norplant (R) trials were made available only recently by the ICMR. The data show that 57.9 per cent of the 1,466 women on whom it was tried, discontinued its use before the end of five years. A significant number (28.5%) did so because of menstrual problems. There were even cases of deep vein thrombosis, arthritis, dimness of vision and infectious hepatitis. In 28 cases, difficulty was experienced with removal. The ICMR scientists dismiss the complications as not very significant, saying that all contraceptives have some side effects and that Norplant offers one more method for women to choose from (ICMR, 1988). According to Medico Friend Circle, an NGO active in the health sector, many women who had undergone trials complained that doctors did not tell them about the nature or the possible side effects of the contraceptive. Proper counselling and adequate medical care was not provided, and even in Delhi, the capital city, several women were lost to follow-up during the controlled trials (Gupta, 2000).

A small study done by the Forum for Women and Health (FFWH), Bombay, to record first person accounts of women who had undergone Norplant trials in Baroda, found that none of the women were aware that they were participating in trials. They were told that it was a new method which would give a contraceptive effect for five years; during this period they did not have to worry about getting pregnant, and they would not have any problems with it. Whether they were suffering from any major or contraindicated illness was not checked. Women's knowledge about their bodies being so limited, an implant inserted with minor surgery in their forearm seems to appeal to them. Those women who eventually had serious problems with the method did not think the method was faulty, but believed that it was all the fault of their own bodies.

The FFWH report points out that in the Baroda trials Muslim women from the state of Uttar Pradesh, who are commonly believed to be reluctant users of contraceptive methods, were especially targeted. At another centre in Thane on the outskirts of Bombay, seven Norplant trial participants were missing, some totally untraceable, who had no permanent address, no work and were vulnerable to pressure because of their circumstances were enrolled for trials. The report concludes that 'in fact, the way the women undergoing the trial are chosen and treated, the whole process seems to be an ultimate violation of the concept of women's choice itself'.

It is clear that the information given to women by providers of the technology is generally limited. The most important message is that it is effective for a certain period; it is safe and has been used a lot in other places, even if it is still in a trial phase. No written materials are provided, though sometimes illustrated brochures are used. Although most technological methods come in packages which contain user information and instructions, they are never handed out. Health and field workers say that this is because the people are illiterate and even too backward to understand what it is written on the inserts. In early 1993, women's group concerned with the health and well-being of Indian women called for a stop to the introduction of Norplant in the National Family Planning Programme before further research demonstrating its safety is done.

### *Sterilization*

Besides abortion, the most common method of contraception used in many developing countries such as India is sterilization, and of this the major share is that of female sterilization. Laparoscopic sterilizations are often done in sub-optimal conditions, either in institutional or mobile settings. In rural areas, camps are organized in temporary locations such as school buildings or some other public facility on special occasions. In these camps, a single surgeon performs 300–500 laparoscopies in 10 hours per day, which works out to one operation every two minutes. With the minimal care that is necessary for such an operation, only a maximum of 50 a day would be possible. There was a report from Kumbakonam that 1,225 women were operated upon in one day. In such a setting, it must be expected that the attitude of the health personnel would be callous. Obviously, follow-up care is not part of such mass programme which provides the facility of sterilization and move on. Often these areas do not have hospitals or clinics where women have problems can go for help (Balasubrahmanyan, 1986).

Most mass sterilization camps are doing far too many sterilizations per day with too few doctors and in inadequate supply of instruments. Ramanathan et al. (1995) note this in their observations at a sub-district level hospital in Kerala. Due to high demand for these services, 48 sterilizations were performed by one surgical team in just over two hours, is clear violation of the regulations. Counselling of women before the operation was inadequate, the surgeon never changed his/her gloves, the linen on the operating tables was never changed and the facilities in the building were grossly insufficient to support post-operation requirements. A study of 9,066 laparoscopies conducted in camps over ten years reported surgical difficulties for 7.9 per cent of the clients, complications for 5.3 per cent, and failure rates of 0.6 per 100 women (Karkal, 1985). Prakash (1984) reports a death rate of 10–12 per 1,00,000 laparoscopic sterilizations, compared to an acceptable figure of 0.25 to 0.5. The Indian Association of Gynaecological Endoscopists issued a strong statement criticizing the way mass sterilization camps are conducted. Some even condemned the way of working of such 'professional laparoscopists' and their 'craze for speed' and the setting of daily targets which have resulted in both 'method failure' as well as medical complications for women (Prakash, 1984).

## Reproductive Technology

Reproductive technologies designed to intervene in the process of human reproduction for the prevention of conception and birth which includes contraceptives as well as methods of pregnancy termination. Since prevention and termination of pregnancy has been analysed under family planning method, therefore, here we turn below to the reproductive technology which helps in aiding or stimulating reproductive process. Reproduction technology is used for assisting reproduction in terms of aiding or stimulating reproduction like artificial insemination, in-vitro fertilization, etc. Reproductive technologies are also used for genetic purposes and for prenatal diagnosis which includes sex detection and sex selection.

Most of the techniques used in assisted reproduction or artificial reproduction were first used in animals such as cows and sheep. Technologies used to assist reproduction are also referred to as 'contraceptive technologies'. They were originally developed to help women with tubal pathologies or in the case of infertility of husband/partner and for idiopathic (unexplained) infertility. These may include such as artificial insemination, in-vitro fertilization, surrogacy, etc.

The uses of technologies for assisting reproduction are extremely controversial; different interest groups in society have contributed to the debates with regard to their own sets of values, norms and interests. Childless individuals and couples see in these technologies a possibility to realize their desire for a child, which they expect to be supported by the providers of the technology and health care facilities. Researchers in human reproduction see it as an opportunity to do fundamental research in studying the processes of conception, the beginnings of human life, and perhaps to manipulate and have more and more of these processes under their control. Critics of these technologies are concerned with their repercussions on society and see in these developments the potential for far-reaching manipulation of the beginning of life, eugenic selection and increase in the control of women's bodies and lives.

### *Artificial Insemination*

Although non-medical artificial insemination has been found for a long time, the first known attempts date back to 1799. The successful use of artificial insemination in humans dates from the 1870s. In artificial insemination a woman is inseminated with a man's sperm, produced after masturbation, without having sexual intercourse. It is a simple procedure entailing sperm being deposited in a woman's vagina close to the cervix. The sperm used could be that of her husband or partner – referred to as artificial insemination by husband's sperm (AIH); or that of a donor, referred to as artificial insemination by a donor sperm (AID). The latter is resorted to when the husband/partner is infertile, has a low sperm count, or a genetic disorder which the parents do not want to pass on to the prospective offspring.

According to infertility specialists, there is a tremendous demand for AID in India. About 500–600 cases of AID are recorded each month. Government hospitals do not provide the facility, thus, private gynaecologists have a booming practice.

Most men are reluctant to even go for semen tests. Requests for AID are accompanied by appeals for utmost secrecy: husband not wanting their wives to know that donor is being used for insemination or the other way around, or parents-in-law requesting their daughter-in-law not be told that their son is sterile. A number of women seem to be concerned that the husband should not be told about his 'lack of manhood'. Women come with their mothers without the knowledge of their husbands and in-laws, because if they do not provide a child they may be deserted. Some doctors, however, do not entertain such requests (Gupta, 2000). Most doctors have a consent form that needs to be signed by both husband and wife before donor sperm is used. Sometimes donor sperm is also sought by couples who have earlier children born with genetic disorders, often due to defects in the husband's sperm. An even more important reason for seeking artificial insemination – AID/AIH – is to increase the chances of getting a male child by inseminating with sperm which has been separated for its X (female) and Y (male) chromosomes and selected for Y-bearing chromosomes (Savara, 1989).

The identity of donors is not recorded as specialists anticipate complications such as paternity suits or blackmail later on.

### *In-Vitro Fertilization*

In-vitro fertilization (IVF) of eggs from mammals began to be developed in the 1930s, however, research in eggs taken from women took long to develop. IVF is at basis of a number of other techniques, making possible other manipulations, such as pre-implantation diagnosis of embryo for genetic disorders and sex selection. Durga Agarwal, born on 3 October 1978, was hailed as the first Indian 'test-tube baby', and second in the world, but her claim to birth through IVF was contested, leading to suicide by Subhas Mukherjee, the doctor who claimed credit for it.

Until the mid-1980s infertility treatment basically consisted of trying to diagnose the cause of infertility, rather than providing a way out. Then came corrective surgery in the form of tuboplasty, lately microscopic tuboplasty. Generally it ended with the doctor giving up and the couple having to resign themselves to their fate, accepting childlessness or going in for adoption wither within the family, or through an adoption agency.

There are over 20 private IVF clinics across the country. However, nowadays a whole range of options exists, from the relatively simple artificial insemination, by husband or donor sperm, to in-vitro fertilization. These services are increasingly offered by private clinics as few government hospitals provide them. In the late 1980s, the All India Institute of Medical Sciences (AIIMS) in New Delhi did offer services for the infertile through its clinic, but stopped after a year. The Institute for Research in Reproduction (IRR) in Mumbai in collaboration with King Edward Memorial (KEM) Hospital has been foremost in research in this field since 1983. But both IRR and KEM Hospital have stopped offering IVF, reportedly due to pressure from feminist groups who pointed out that most clinics practising IVF also indulged in sex determination and sex selection. Now, private gynaecologists are providing these services. The number of patients coming for assisted conception is growing phenomenally. IVF treatments are extremely expensive, anything from ₹ 50,000–10,00,000 depending on the number of attempts necessary. As there is no system of health insurance and government hospitals do not provide the facility, people have to pay for it themselves (Gupta, 2000).

### *Surrogacy*

Surrogacy is a method of assisted reproduction. The word 'surrogate' originates from Latin word 'surrogatus' (substitution) – to act in place of. The term 'surrogacy' is used when a woman carries a pregnancy and gives birth to a baby for another women. In India, in the joint family system surrogate mothering (social, not biological) is common; widowed family members and older daughters also 'mother' children. The social role fulfilment is stressed rather than the biological process of child birth. The first known case of technological surrogacy reported by Sucha Menon concerned a childless couple from Mumbai who were both infertile and thus opted for surrogacy. Menon asks what the repercussions of renting a womb are likely to be in a society which puts self-sacrificing motherhood on a pedestal.

Thirty-year old Nirmala from Chandigarh caused uproar when she announced her decision to bear a child for an infertile couple for ₹ 50,000. The womb is used to earn money. Nirmala was threatened with action under Suppression of Immoral Traffic Act. Subsequently, she filed a law suit seeking legal sanction for her action and threatened to commit sati if her husband dies for lack of medical help.

Surrogacy is gaining popularity as this may be the only method for a couple to have their own child and also because adoption process may be a long drawn out process. A growing number of women in Anand district of Gujarat, the home of Amul and the milk producers' cooperatives, is emerging as a magnet for childless couples. Eighteen women have offered themselves as surrogate mothers. These women, mostly from the lower middle income group, are under the care of Dr Nayana H. Patel, a gynaecologist using the IVF method. She said at her hospital here: 'Women preferring to become surrogate mothers are briefed (they are told) they will have to hand over the child ...' Jyotsana Patel, 30, preparing to become a surrogate mother for a third time, said: 'I opted to rent out my womb to a childless couple ... I also got to make good money.' Asked why childless couples from the US and UK and other parts of world and India prefer this method over adoption, the doctor said they keep genes and ethnic reasons in mind. Cost is a key factor too: it is much cheaper in India. According to her, agencies abroad charge $30,000 and the surrogate mother is given $15,000. She said in India surrogate mothers get between ₹ 1 lakh and 2 lakhs (*The Hindu*, 2 March 2006).

At the moment technologies in the field of assisted reproduction affect only a small section number of people, although they are proliferating at a very rapid pace. In India there is no law on AID or IVF and no body of experts to supervise the ethics of business or to certify the institutions.

The reporting in the media has wither been a glorification of the success stories of conceptive technologies, or critical in terms of their effects in a country with an already large population. Opposition to technologies used in assisted reproduction from a feminist perspective is less known. Lakshi Lingam, while doing a print media analysis, argues that it is crucial to view contraceptive technologies as links in the same chain (as sex-determination technologies) based on uniform ideologies of 'abusing, disrespecting, manipulating and exploiting women as 'objects'. She says that IVF technology is anti-woman for it is set within the ideological structure of 'marriage', 'children within wedlock', 'the supremacy of biological motherhood' and it reinforces fertility as an important indicator of women's status (Lingam, 1990).

The extraordinary and rapid advance of biological and genetic technology is going to give rise to new and complicated issues in the future that were unknown in our country. The status of children born by artificial insemination, or the legal status of surrogate mother, is just some of the issues that might come to the courts in the future.

## Conclusion

Non-recognition of health as a citizen's social right only underscores the low priority it has had in the shaping of public policy. With few exceptions, most laws in India make no distinction between health and female in the area of health. Some laws, taking note of the specific features of our society, are however, protectionist in nature. The protectionist kind of laws would include Maternity Benefit Act, Medical Termination of Pregnancy Act, etc.

We already have the misuse of technology in pre-natal diagnostic techniques to determine the sex of the child foetus and then its selective abortion. Amniocentesis is carried on in parts of the country despite legislation in certain states to regulate the tests.

There are certain issues related to women's health which might come to the courts in future. Legislation in itself cannot, however, curb deep-rooted prejudices and traditional customs that are detrimental to women's well-being.

## References

Balasubrahmanyan, V. (1986), *Contraception as if Women Mattered: A Critique of Family Planning*, Bombay: Centre for Education and Documentation.

Bhatia, Jagdish C. (1988), *A Study of Maternal Mortality in Anantapur District, Andhra Pradesh, India*, Bangalore: Indian Institute of Management.

Chhabra, Rami and Sheel C. Nuna (1994), *Abortion in India: An Overview*, New Delhi: Ford Foundation.

Forum for Women's Health (FFWH) (undated), *Anti-fertility Vaccine*, Bombay: Media Packet.

——. *Norplant: Reflections on Some Experiences*, Bombay.

George, Sabu (2006), 'Millions of Missing Girls: From Fetal Sexing to High Technology Sex Selection in India', *Prental Diagnosis*, Vol. 26, Issue 7, July, pp. 604–609.

Government of India (1966), *Report of the Committee to Study the Question of Legislation of Abortion*, Ministry of Health and Family Planning, p. 40.

Grand, A. Le (1990), Medical and Users' Aspects of RU 486 with Particular Emphasis on its Use in Third World Countries in WEMOS, pp. 19–28.

——. (1992), 'The Abortion Pill: A Solution for Unsafe Abortions in Developing Countries?', *Social Science and Medicine*, Vol. 35, No. 6, pp. 767–76.

Gupta, Jyotsna Agnihotri (2000), *New Reproductive Technologies, Women's Health and Autonomy: Freedom or Dependency?*, New Delhi: Sage Publications.

Gupta, M.C. (2002), *Health and Law: A Guide for Professionals and Activists*, New Delhi: Kanishka Publishers.

Indian Council of Medical Research (ICMR) (1988), *Overview of Trends in Maternal Mortality*, Report of a Workshop, New Delhi.

Karkal, M. (1985), *Family Planning in India: A Critical Appraisal*, Meeting of the National Committee for Natural Family Planning, 3–7 November, Washington, DC.

Lingam, Lakshmi (1990), 'New Reproductive Technologies in India: A Print Media Analysis, Reproductive and Genetic Engineering', *International Feminist Analysis*, Vol. 3, No. 1, pp. 13–21.

MoHFW (Ministry of Health and Family Welfare) (1992), *Action Plan for Revamping the Family Welfare Programme in India*, New Delhi.

Nair, Amrita (1991), 'The Variety of Ways', *Free Press Journal*, 13 January.

Population Council (1990), *Norplant Contraceptive Subdermal Implants: Manual for Clinicians*, New York.

Prakash, Padma (1984), 'Use of Laparoscopy for Sterilization', *Economic and Political Weekly*, 17 March, pp. 453–54.

——. (1986), 'Injectable Contraceptives (NET-EN) in the Context of the Family Planning Programme', paper presented at a Workshop organized by the Campaign against Long Acting Contraceptives (CALAC), 10 August.

Ramanathan, M. et al. (1995), 'Quality of Care in Laparoscopic Sterilization Camps: Observations from Kerala, India', *Reproductive Health Matters*, No. 6, November, pp. 84–93.

Ramaseshan, Geeta (1999), 'Some Reflections on Women and Health Under the Law', in Swapna Mukhopadhyay (ed.), *In the Name of Justice: Women and Law in Society*, New Delhi: Manohar Publications.

Rao, K. Bhaskar (1988), 'Maternal Mortality in India', paper presented at the Annual Meeting of the Indian Medical Association, New Delhi.

Reddy, P.H. (1992), 'Maternal Mortality in Karnataka', Draft Paper, Bangalore: Population Centre.

Savara, M. (1989), 'New Reproductive Technology and Women', paper presented at the International Science Policy Foundation Meeting, XIX All India Sociological Conference at Hissar and New Delhi.

*The Times of India* (2006), March 28.

Toubia (1991) quoted in M.E. Hunt (1992), 'RU 486/PG and Ethics: Women's Moral Property, Not for Sale', *Conscience*, Vol. XIII, No. 1, pp. 3–10.

World Bank (1996), *Improving Women's Health in India*, Washington, DC.

World Health Organisation (WHO) (1946), Constitution of the WHO, Reprinted in *Basic Documents*, 37th edition, Geneva.

# 6 Women and Ethics in Medicine

## Historical Perspective and Contemporary Concern

Numerous indicators reflect a growing interest in ethical issues in medical and health care. Increasingly media coverage includes discussion of ethical issues surrounding such developments as has been the case with reproductive technologies such as surrogate motherhood, cloning of human beings, etc. Moreover, professional organizations are devoting more time at their meetings and more space in their publications to discussion of ethical issues (Gottlieb, Burdine and McLeory, 1987). Against this background one night suspect an equivalent development of sociological interest in medical ethics. This is so because many issues in medical ethics are sociological in nature and have aroused considerable interest. For example, work in the area of medical care ethics, particularly work focusing on the rights and duties of medical professionals and patients, bears directly on the evolving nature of the doctor-patient relationship (Stacey, 1985). Ethical analysis of medical and health care public policy has significant implication for such macro-sociological issues as equality in access to care and the role of the professions in determining the availability of medical and health care services (Mechanic, 1979).

A review of recent medical sociology works reveals some coverage of an array of ethical issues in medical and health care (Mechanic, 1983; Susser, Watson and Hopper, 1985; Mechanic and Aiken, 1986; Simmons and Canio, 1979). Much of this has focused on micro-ethical issues, such as the doctor-patient relationship and treatment decisions for critically ill patients (Crane, 1975). More recently there has been an extension to societally focused issues, such as the rationing of medical care (Mechanic, 1979). Lesser attention has been devoted to exploring ethical issues in the interactions between institutions and professionals to studying the dynamic relationships between the professions and society (Freidson, 1970). Some sociological attention also has been given to the rise and current interest in bioethics (Fox, 1974). The number of specific medical and health issues that have received ethical analysis is very large; they include such topics as death and dying, kidney dialysis, organ transplantation, clinical research, genetic counselling and screening, decision to extend or terminate life support system, allocation of scarce medical resources, cost containment, and ethical issues in the development of for-profit hospitals.

In India, not much work has been done on medical ethics, however, Desai (1988) tried to see the medical ethics in the continuity of indigenous and classical folk traditions. Wig (1985) discussed the forced population control measures as a medical and ethical issue. Desai and Chand (2007) lamented on the lacunae and absence of laws specifically with the duties of health facilities and personnel to provide medical treatment in emergency cases. Sriram et al. (1991) and Minocha (2010) have studied the discourse of informed consent in medical ethics along with field observation. There is not much work at the theoretical and empirical levels which has been done on the medical ethics, particularly in the Indian context.

The purpose of this chapter is to provide a historical overview of the developments in the field of ethics concerning medicine and health. The discourse also focuses on morals and ethics. We summarize major principles around which much of ethics debates concerning medical and health care have been organized. Following this, the chapter connects the medical ethics in India with the contemporary concern of women.

## I

## History of Medical Ethics

Since the beginning of human history, concern for medical ethics has been expressed in the form of laws, decrees, assumptions and oaths prepared for or by physicians. Among the oldest of these are the Code of Hammurabi in Babylonia (approximately 1750 BCE), Egyptian papyri, Indian and Chinese writings, and early Greek writers, mostly Hippocrates (lived between 460 and 377 BCE). Early medical ethical codes were written by individuals or by small groups of people, usually physicians. The oath of Hippocrates is considered historically to be the first such code written in an organized and logical way which describes the proper relationships between physician and patient. During the Middle Ages, other medical codes were written. In recent times, Thomas Precival's writings, disseminated in 1803, represent one of the first ethical codes in the United States and the Western World (Lustig et al., 1993).

Beginning in the second half of the 19th century medical organizations began writing codes of medical ethics. The first ethics code of the American Medical Association (AMA) was published in 1847. This was the first ethical code of a professional organization which outlined the rights of patients and caregivers. In the 19th century, medicine along with university teaching, law and the ministry underwent professionalization. The medical profession succeeded, after prolonged agitation, in getting recognition for their status and prestige, in 1858 when the Act creating the General Medical Council was passed in the UK. Initially, the Medical Councils of developed countries paid almost exclusive attention to reducing competition from outside and within. Thus, traditional practitioners and quacks were forcibly eliminated in the later part of the 19th century. Elaborate codes were made to restrict or eliminate unhealthy competition within the profession. Entry to the profession was restricted by getting control over the medical education and registration of doctors. To these were gradually added the internal regulations or disciplinary procedures to curb misuse of power detrimental to patients' well-being.

The World Health Organization (WHO) issued the Declaration of Geneva in 1948. This is the first worldwide ethical code and is modelled after the oath of Hippocrates. Many other medical organizations throughout the world have issued medical ethical codes.

## Meaning of Ethics

Ethics involve normative questions, reasoning, and decision – for example, how one should act or that ought one do, both as a moral ideal and in an actual situation? Normative ethics, as a discipline, is not synonymous with law or the social sciences.

## Theories of Ethics

Ethics is the branch of philosophy that has traditionally concerned itself with examining the worth or value of conduct, with developing and defending views on what might be meant by a 'worthwhile' and with how such a life could be led. Different ethical traditions have developed separate – and conflicting – views on the purpose of ethics (metaethical views) and the on the kind of ethics in which we should actually engage (normative views). In particular, western philosophy has been profoundly shaped by three theories of ethics: Aristotelianism, deontology and utilitarianism. Each of these three theories can in turn be seen as essentially a product of the times in which it was originally born. These theories are based on trying to determine:

- What is meant by leading a good or virtuous life (the focus particularly of Aristotelianism)?
- What kinds of duty or obligation we owe each other (the focus particularly of deontology)?
- How we might take account of consequences when deciding a particular course of action (the focus especially of utilitarianism)?

### *Aristotelianism*

Aristotle's ethics are representative of ethical theories that aim to work out what a good (moral) life might mean and how the development of such life can be encouraged. He attempted to do this by looking at the nature of the world and the individuals within it in order to assess what being virtuous might mean. For this reason Aristotle is frequently thought of as an empiricist. In viewing the world, he argued that we become virtuous by performing virtuous actions. What is most important is not simply the identification of the mean (the virtuous) in all aspects of human actions. It is the idea that, through reflection and contemplation, we should develop our lives so that we know how to act virtuously (or morally). We thus become more morally expert, and the consequent performance of virtuous actions determining, what it means to lead to the worthwhile (good) life.

### *Deontology*

Immanuel Kant developed ideas representative of deontology – thinking based on the notion that we owe each other particular duties or obligations. Kant claimed the existence of a reality independent of our experience. Part of his justification for his claim lay in his analysis of our experience as humans. We live in a world subject to scientific laws of causation, yet we retain freedom of will, having the capacity to act morally or otherwise. Out moral choices must, therefore, be framed within an independent reality. Kant argued that reasons exist independently of experience and that the right use of reason is directed towards moral ends. Reasons move us to act out of duty for its own sake and independently of any thought about the consequences. How, then, is the difficulty to overcome? One way (which of course the strict deontologist could not accept) is to allow that consideration of consequences to play an important part in making moral decisions. This leads to the third ethical tradition to be considered – utilitarianism.

### *Utilitarianism*

According to J.S. Mill careful thought needs to be given to the consequences of any action, and if those consequences are likely to adverse for some, the reason for the action must be robust. Utility, or the greatest happiness principle, holds that actions are right in proportion as they tend to promote happiness, and wrong as they tend to produce the reverse of happiness. By happiness means intended pleasure, and the absence of pain; by unhappiness, pain, and the privation of pleasure (Mill, 1962). Utilitarianism and consequentialist ethical theory in general corresponds with a belief held by many that whereas there are important moral duties, action simply for the sake of duty, whatever the consequences, is problematic. In addition, a deliberation about consequences may well include thoughts about the level of 'happiness' or 'unhappiness' likely to accrue from a particular course of action.

## Ethical and Moral Discourse

In the ethnographic terms, moral processes differ in a fundamental way from ethical discourse. Whereas moral experience is always about practical engagements in a particular local world, a cultural space that carries political, economic and psychological specificity –

a view from somewhere and actions and reactions that are partisan – ethical discourse is a globally elaborated abstract articulation of and debate over translocal values. It strives for an acontextual universality and objectivity – a view from nowhere. Ethical discourse is generated out of and applied in local worlds, however, so that it gets taken up in moral processes that are inseparable from local elations and conditions. The institutions, relationships and lived experiences that serve ethical deliberations are themselves grounded, of course, in the oral processes of local worlds, so that in actual practice, the distinction has blurred boundaries with overlapping components. But for heuristic purposes it is still useful to draw the distinction between local and moral processes that are inseparable from local relations and conditions and ethical discourse that brings, or at least aspires to, a translocal perspective (Kleinman, 2004).

The other side of the duality is that ethics can be (and all-too-frequently are) irrelevant to local moral worlds. Thus, structural positioning of poverty and wealth systematically distributes health and health care resources inequitably as part of what defines the moral reality of a local world. To talk about universal ethical formulations of justice and equity, without beginning with the local moral condition of real people who experience the systematic injustices of higher rates of ill health and fewer health care resources owing to their positioning in local social structures of power is to make those formulations utopian and irrelevant to the local world (Daniels et al., 1999). When, for example, informed consent in bioethics is made into the overriding ethical condition of international health research, say in vaccine trials of HIV in impoverished African villages where few people are literate and there is no equivalent in local knowledge of ideas of randomised controlled trials, placebo controls, or perhaps even individual autonomy in deciding about participation in a community-wide activity, while the systematic injustice in the global economy that has deepened these people's poverty and suffering via structural adjustment programmes and the local conditions of absence of the most basic health care resources to treat AIDS are also absent from ethical discourse, then application of the ethical in the local setting of the oral is highly suspect (cf. Farmer, 1999).

## Theoretical and Methodological Perspectives in Ethics

The territory of ethics – the examination and discussion of the values underpinning conduct – is largely conceptual, and in the case of many of the concepts discussed in ethics, there is a large degree of dispute, or contestedness. Some philosophers have attempted to suggest that value ('ought') judgements have a status roughly equivalent to those concerning empirical fact, that in asserting, for example, 'killing is wrong', someone is suggesting an undeniable truth. Aristotle, Kant and Mill are very important representatives of philosophers attempting normative moral projects. In more recent times, contemporary thinkers viewing health care have tried to suggest that there are important principles that should underlie work in this field of activity. Among others, Beauchamp and Childress (1994) and Gillon (1994) have suggested the following principles that are particularly important for health care workers:

- *Autonomy:* It is the capacity to be in charge yourself of your actions and your destiny. The principle of respect for autonomy asserts that we have a moral obligation to allow this capacity to individuals to the extent that it does not infringe on the equal rights of others. The obligation to respect the autonomy of others – for example, patients or clients – to the extent that this is compatible with the autonomy of all who are likely to be affected by the action being considered.
- *Beneficence:* This is frequently regarded as a moral obligation that ought to be held by health care workers and clearly connects with beneficence. The ethical commitment in health care to produce benefit for patients or clients.
- *Non-maleficence:* The obligation not to harm patients or clients, closely linked to the previous principles, because any given action has the potential to result in both benefit and harm. The obligation on health care professionals is to ensure that the balance is always in favour of benefit in any given situation.
- *Justice:* The obligation to act fairly when dealing with competing claims to do with, for example, resources or rights.

Importantly, the above four principles are prima facie, which means that each is binding unless it conflicts with another, in which case a choice must be made between the competing principles as to which one should be followed. Those who support the four principles argue that whereas they cannot yield a definitive ethical judgement in all health care situations, they do provide a framework for considering, and reasoning about obligations.

Medical ethics is an area of applied ethics concerned with health and illness and health care and medical care. Ethics applied to health care and medicine have a number of roles to play and a number of limitations (Beauchamp and Childress, 1983). Most people involved in medical ethics would agree that it is a useful but rather imprecise 'diagnostic' and 'prescriptive' tool when brought to bear on real-life situations. 'Moral action guides' but seldom offers ready solutions to the hard choices that confront providers, patients, or policy makers. This is so, in part, because medical ethics most often deal with dilemmas in which no set of moral reasons for a given view or action is obviously the correct one.

## II
## Medical Ethics in India

The beginnings of recorded medical practice in India date back to the advent of Aryan invaders. Much useful information is also found in the seminal ayurvedic classics *Caraka Samhita, Susruta Samhita* and *Bhela Samhita* (around 600 BC). In these classics, ethical principles were enunciated and steps taken to ensure that they were followed. Teacher and student were reminded that the profession existed for the welfare of the patient. Whilst fair compensation was not frowned upon, the physician was constantly reminded that the primary goal was not fortune for self and family but the care of the sick. The healthy human body is essential to the realization of life's tasks, including the ethical. Seeking health was a religious obligation. Ayurveda was created before the creation of the world, so that the potential for protection of health and removal of disease were built into the act of creation. Ethical laws were natural laws, and the ayurvedic world-view was a part of the Hindu conception of humanity and its place in the universe.

The advent of the Portuguese, French and, most significantly, the British into India witnessed in the system of medicine that continues to dominate the subcontinent. The officers of the Indian Medical Service introduced the principles of medicine and western concept of medical ethics. To this day, discussion on ethics in India starts with the enumeration of the principles of beneficence, non-malevolence, autonomy and justice (Pandya, 2000). Questions about medical ethics in India interact with local customs and tradition in everyday practice. Unusual occurrences may be resolved by a reference to mythology or folklore. This is not to suggest that Indian medicine does not address the problems of ethics. They are intertwined in medical texts, and mythical figures are seen as models of exemplary ethical behaviour. Ethical solutions may be inferred and derived from scriptural texts. This is particularly so in the context of modern and recent medical technologies, with which medicine in India has no prior contact (Desai, 1988).

In India, the formal process of medical profession began in 1912 when the Bombay Medical Act was passed. This was followed in 1914 by the Madras Medical Registration Act, Bengal Medical Act and the like. In 1933, the Indian Medical Council Act brought higher education in medicine under the purview of a national level medical council. After independence, separate national and state level councils were created for allopathy, homeopathy and the Indian System of Medicine (ISM). The Medical Council of India, under the Medical Council Act, 1956, in 2002 made the regulations relating to the professional conduct, etiquette and ethics for registered medical practitioners. We will discuss them in the ensuing pages.

## Functioning of Medical Council

The national level council has control and supervision over medical education whereas the state councils maintain registers of doctors and have powers to punish doctors whose conduct was found to be unethical. Under the Act, the Medical Council is empowered to hold an enquiry of any registered doctor suo moto (on its own) or any complaint made to it. Thus, the Medical Council can act against the erring doctor even if no complaint is filled by the patient(s).

Further, the Medical Council has the power to punish those doctors who are found guilty of much misconduct in a properly held enquiry. Accordingly, it can warn a doctor, or can temporarily or permanently remove his/her name from the register. But, the Council has no power to award compensation to the patient. When there are persistent reports of unethical practices in the profession (e.g., organ trade, commission practices), the Council cannot advance a pretext that there is no specific complaint filed. The Council has suo moto power to investigate. This also provides scope to patients' organizations and social organizations in filing complaints and in pressurizing the medical councils to play a more active role.

## Importance of Medical Ethics

Medical ethics are not merely a moral code but a legally sanctioned code of conduct acceptable within the medical profession. This does not mean that morality or moral theories do not influence medical ethics, but medical ethics must be understood, analysed and practised from a rational standpoint. This rational component of professional conduct is legally codified under the code of medical ethics of the legally constituted Medical Council with which all qualified medical practitioners must be registered.

The registrations as well as the conduct as per the code of ethics are essential because, 'doctors use technical skills and expertise which the untrained person does not possess. Possessing these skills gives him great power over his patients who by the very fact of being patients are dependent, ill and vulnerable. In caring for his patients, a doctor makes a series of judgements and decisions which patients have the right to expect are made fairly in the light of the doctor's knowledge and experience' (British Medical Association, 1988). Thus, although the code of medical ethics is for the self-regulation of the profession, it is there in order to fulfil certain rights and expectations of the patient. In a nutshell, the code describes the doctor's duties towards the patient. If these rights are not fulfilled or duties are not performed, then the doctor in question loses his or her right to be part of the profession.

## Code of Ethics Regulations, 2002 (amended up to December 2010)

In exercise of the powers conferred under section 20A read with section 33(m) of the Indian Medical Council Act, 1956 (102 of 1956), the Medical Council of India, with the previous approval of the Central Government, has made the following regulations relating to the professional conduct, etiquette and ethics for registered medical practitioners. These regulations may be called the Indian Medical Council (Professional Conduct, Etiquette and Ethics) Regulations, 2002.

## 1. CODE OF MEDICAL ETHICS

### *(a) Declaration*

Each applicant, at the time of making an application for registration under the provisions of the Act, shall be provided a copy of the declaration and shall submit a duly signed declaration. The applicant shall also certify that he/she had read and agreed to abide by the same.

### *(b) Duties and responsibilities of the physician in general*

1.1 Character of physician(doctors with qualification of MBBS or MBBS with post-graduate degree/diploma or with equivalent qualification in any medical discipline):

1.1.1 A physician shall uphold the dignity and honour of his/her profession.

1.1.2 The prime object of the medical profession is to render service to humanity; reward or financial gain is a subordinate consideration. Whosoever chooses his/her profession, assumes the obligation to conduct himself/herself in accordance with its ideals. A physician should be an upright man/woman, instructed in the art of healings. He/she shall keep himself pure in character and be diligent in caring for the sick; he/she should be modest, sober, patient, prompt in discharging his duty without anxiety; conducting himself/herself with propriety in his/her profession and in all the actions of his life.

1.1.3 No person other than a doctor having qualification recognized by Medical Council of India (MCI) and registered with Medical Council of India/State Medical Council (s) is allowed to practise modern system of medicine or surgery. A person obtaining qualification in any other system of medicine is not allowed to practise modern system of medicine in any form.

1.2 Maintaining good medical practice:

1.2.1 The principal objective of the medical profession is to render service to humanity with full respect for the dignity of profession and man. Physicians should merit the confidence of patients entrusted to their care, rendering to each a full measure of service and devotion. They should also try continuously to improve medical knowledge and skills and should make available to their patients and colleagues the benefits of their professional attainments. The physician should practise methods of healing founded on scientific basis and should not associate professionally with anyone who violates this principle. The honoured ideals of the medical profession imply that the responsibilities of the physician extend not only to individuals but also to society.

1.2.2 Membership in medical society: For the advancement of his/her profession, a physician should affiliate with associations and societies of allopathic medical professions and involve actively in the functioning of such bodies.

1.2.3 A physician should also participate in professional meetings as part of continuing medical education programmes, for at least 30 hours every five years, organized by reputed professional academic bodies or any other authorized organizations. The compliance of this requirement shall be informed regularly to MCI or the State Medical Councils as the case may be.

1.3 Maintenance of medical records:

1.3.1 Every physician shall maintain the medical records pertaining to his/her indoor patients for a period of three years from the date of commencement of the treatment in a standard proforma laid down by the MCI.

1.3.2. If any request is made for medical records either by the patients/authorized attendant or legal authorities involved, the same may be duly acknowledged and documents shall be issued within the period of 72 hours.

1.3.3 A registered medical practitioner shall also maintain a Register of Medical Certificates giving full details of certificates issued. When issuing a medical certificate he/she shall always enter the identification marks of the patient and keep a copy of the certificate. He/she shall not omit to record the signature and/or thumb mark, address and at least one identification mark of the patient on the medical certificates or report.

1.3.4 Efforts shall be made to computerize medical records for quick retrieval.

1.4 Display of registration numbers:

1.4.1 Every physician shall display the registration number accorded to him/her by the State Medical Council/MCI in his clinic and in all his prescriptions, certificates, and money receipts given to his/her patients.

1.4.2 Physicians shall display as suffix to their names only recognized medical degrees or such certificates/diplomas and memberships/honours which confer professional knowledge or recognize any exemplary qualification/achievements.

1.5 Use of generic names of drugs: Every physician should, as far as possible, prescribe drugs with generic names and he/she shall ensure that there is a rational prescription and use of drugs.

1.6 Highest quality assurance in patient care: Every physician should aid in safeguarding the profession against admission to it of those who are deficient in moral character or education. Physician shall not employ in connection with his/her professional practice any attendant who is neither registered nor enlisted under the Medical Acts in force and shall not permit such persons to attend, treat or perform operations upon patients wherever professional discretion or skill is required.

1.7 Exposure of unethical conduct: A physician should expose, without fear or favour, incompetent or corrupt, dishonest or unethical conduct on the part of members of the profession.

1.8 Payment of professional services: The physician, engaged in the practice of medicine, shall always give priority to the interests of patients. The personal financial interests of a physician should not conflict with the medical interests of patients. A physician should announce his/her fees before rendering service and not after the operation or treatment is under way. Remuneration received for such services should be in the form and amount specifically announced to the patient at the time the service is rendered. It is unethical to enter into a contract of 'no cure no payment'. Physician rendering service on behalf of the state shall refrain from anticipating or accepting any consideration.

1.9 Evasion of legal restrictions: The physician shall observe the laws of the country in regulating the practice of medicine and shall also not assist others to evade such laws. He/she should be cooperative in observance and enforcement of sanitary laws and regulations in the interest of public health. A physician should observe the provisions of the State Acts like Drugs and Cosmetics Act, 1940; Pharmacy Act, 1948; Narcotic Drugs and Psychotropic Substances Act, 1985; Medical Termination of Pregnancy Act, 1971; Transplantation of Human Organ Act, 1994; Mental Health Act, 1987; Environmental Protection Act, 1986; Pre-natal Sex Determination Test Act, 1994; Drugs and Magic Remedies (Objectionable Advertisement) Act, 1954; Persons with Disabilities (Equal Opportunities and Full Participation) Act, 1995; Bio-Medical Waste (Management and Handling) Rules, 1998 and such other Acts, rules, and regulations made by the Central/State Governments or local administrative bodies or any other relevant Act relating to the protection and promotion of public health.

## 2. DUTIES OF PHYSICIANS TO THEIR PATIENTS

2.1 Obligations to the sick:

2.1.1 Though a physician is not bound to treat each and every person asking his/her services, he/she should not only be ever ready to respond to the calls of the sick and the injured, but should be mindful of the high character of his/her mission and the responsibility he discharges in the course of his/her professional duties. In his/her treatment, he/she should never forget that the health and the lives of those entrusted to his/her care depend on his/her skill and attention. A physician should endeavour to add to the comfort of the sick by making his/her visits at the hour indicated to the patients. A physician advising a patient to seek service of another physician is acceptable, however, in case of emergency a physician must treat the patient. No physician shall arbitrarily refuse treatment to a patient. However, for good reason, when a patient is suffering from an ailment which is not within the range of experience of the treating physician, the physician may refuse treatment and refer the patient to another physician.

2.1.2 Medical practitioner having any incapacity detrimental to the patient or which can affect his/her performance vis-à-vis the patient is not permitted to practise his/her profession

2.2 Patience, delicacy and secrecy: Patience and delicacy should characterize the physician. Confidences concerning individual or domestic life entrusted by patients to a physician and defects in the disposition or character of patients observed during medical attendance should never be revealed unless their revelation is required by the laws of the state. Sometimes, however, a physician must determine whether his/her duty to society requires him/her to employ knowledge, obtained through confidence as a physician, to protect a healthy person against a communicable disease to which he/she is about to be exposed. In such instance, the physician should act as he/she would wish another to act toward one of his/her own family in like circumstances.

2.3 Prognosis: The physician should neither exaggerate nor minimize the gravity of a patient's condition. He/she should ensure himself/herself that the patient, his/her relatives or his/her responsible friends have such knowledge of the patient's condition as will serve the best interests of the patient and the family.

2.4 The patient must not be neglected: A physician is free to choose whom he/she will serve. He/she should, however, respond to any request for his assistance in an emergency. Once having undertaken a case, the physician should not neglect the patient, nor should he/she withdraw from the case without giving adequate notice to the patient and his family. Provisionally or fully registered medical practitioner shall not wilfully commit an act of negligence that may deprive his/her patient or patients from necessary medical care.

2.5 Engagement for an obstetric case: When a physician, who has been engaged to attend an obstetric case, is absent and another is sent for and delivery accomplished, the acting physician is entitled to his/her professional fees, but should secure the patient's consent to resign on the arrival of the physician engaged.

## 3. DUTIES OF PHYSICIAN IN CONSULTATION

3.1 Unnecessary consultations should be avoided:

3.1.1 However, in case of serious illness and in doubtful or difficult conditions, the physician should request consultation, but under any circumstances such consultation should be justifiable and in the interest of the patient only and not for any other consideration.

3.1.2 Consulting pathologists/radiologists or asking for any other diagnostic lab investigation should be done judiciously and not in a routine manner.

3.2 Consultation for patient's benefit: In every consultation, the benefit to the patient is of foremost importance. All physicians engaged in the case should be frank with the patient and his attendants.

3.3 Punctuality in consultation: Utmost punctuality should be observed by a physician in making themselves available for consultations.

3.4 Statement to patient after consultation:

3.4.1 All statements to the patient or his/her representatives should take place in the presence of the consulting physicians, except as otherwise agreed. The disclosure of the opinion to the patient or his/her relatives or friends shall rest with the medical attendant.

3.4.2 Differences of opinion should not be divulged unnecessarily but when there is irreconcilable difference of opinion the circumstances should be frankly and impartially explained to the patient or his/her relatives or friends. It would be opened to them to seek further advice as they so desire.

3.5 Treatment after consultation: No decision should restrain the attending physician from making such subsequent variations in the treatment if any unexpected change occurs, but at the next consultation, reasons for the variations should be discussed/explained. The same privilege, with its obligations, belongs to the consultant when sent for in an emergency during the absence of attending physician. The attending physician may prescribe medicine at any time for the patient, whereas the consultant may prescribe only in case of emergency or as an expert when called for.

3.6 Patients referred to specialists: When a patient is referred to a specialist by the attending physician, a case summary of the patient should be given to the specialist, who should communicate his opinion in writing to the attending physician.

3.7 Fees and other charges:

3.7.1 A physician shall clearly display his/her fees and other charges on the board of his/her chamber and/or the hospitals he/she is visiting. Prescription should also make clear if the physician himself/herself dispensed any medicine.

3.7.2 A physician shall write his/her name and designation in full along with registration particulars in his/her prescription letter head.

*Note:* In government hospital where the patient load is heavy, the name of the prescribing doctor must be written below his/her signature.

## 4. RESPONSIBILITIES OF PHYSICIANS TO EACH OTHER

4.1 A physician should consider it as a pleasure and privilege to render gratuitous service to all other physicians and their immediate family members.

4.2 Conduct in consultation: In consultations, no insincerity, rivalry or envy should be indulged in. All due respect should be observed towards the physician-in-charge of the case and no statement or remark be made, which would impair the confidence reposed in him/her. For this purpose no discussion should be carried on in the presence of the patient or his/her representatives.

4.3 Consultant not to take charge of the case: When a physician has been called for consultation, the consultant should normally not take charge of the case, especially on the solicitation of the patient or friends. The consultant shall not criticize the referring physician. He/she shall discuss the diagnosis treatment plan with the referring physician.

4.4 Appointment of substitute: Whenever a physician requests another physician to attend his/her patients during his/her temporary absence from his/her practice, professional courtesy requires the acceptance of such appointment only when he/she has the capacity to discharge the additional responsibility along with his/her other duties. The physician acting under such an appointment should give the utmost consideration to the interests and reputation of the absent physician and all such patients should be restored to the care of the latter upon his/her return.

4.5 Visiting another physician's case: When it becomes the duty of a physician occupying an official position to see and report upon an illness or injury, he/she should communicate to the physician in attendance so as to give him/her an option of being present. The medical officer/physician occupying an official position should avoid remarks upon the diagnosis or the treatment that has been adopted.

## 5. DUTIES OF PHYSICIAN TO THE PUBLIC AND TO THE PARAMEDICAL PROFESSION

5.1 Physicians as citizens: Physicians, as good citizens, and possessed of special training, should disseminate advice on public health issues. They should play their part in enforcing the laws of the community and in sustaining the institutions that advance the interests of humanity. They should particularly co-operate with the authorities in the administration of sanitary/public health laws and regulations.

5.2 Public and community health: Physicians, especially those engaged in public health work, should enlighten the public concerning quarantine regulations and measures for the prevention of epidemic and communicable diseases. At all times the physician should notify the constituted public health authorities of every case of communicable disease under his/her care, in accordance with the laws, rules and regulations of the health authorities. When an epidemic occurs a physician should not abandon his/her duty for fear of contracting the disease himself/herself.

5.3 Pharmacists/nurses: Physicians should recognize and promote the practice of different paramedical services such as pharmacy and nursing as professions and should seek their cooperation wherever required.

## 6. UNETHICAL ACTS

A physician shall not aid or abet or commit any of the following acts which shall be construed as unethical:

6.1 Advertising

6.1.1 Soliciting of patients directly or indirectly, by a physician, by a group of physicians or by institutions or organizations is unethical. A physician shall not make use of him/her (or his/her name) as subject of any form or manner of advertising or publicity through any mode either alone or in conjunction with others which is of such a character as to invite attention to him/her or to his/her professional position, skill, qualification, achievements, attainments, specialities, appointments, associations, affiliations or honours and/or of such character as would ordinarily result in his/her self-aggrandizement. A physician shall not give to any person, whether for compensation or otherwise, any approval, recommendation, endorsement, certificate, report or statement with respect of any drug, medicine, nostrum remedy, surgical, or therapeutic article, apparatus or appliance or any commercial product or article with respect of any property, quality or use thereof or any test, demonstration or trial thereof, for use in connection with his name, signature, or photograph in any form or manner of advertising through any mode nor shall he/she boast of cases, operations, cures or remedies or permit the publication of report thereof through any mode. A medical practitioner is however permitted to make a formal announcement in press regarding the following:

1. On starting practice.
2. On change of type of practice.
3. On changing address.
4. On temporary absence from duty.
5. On resumption of another practice.
6. On succeeding to another practice.
7. Public declaration of charges.

6.1.2 Printing of self photograph, or any such material of publicity in the letter head or on sign board of the consulting room or any such clinical establishment shall be regarded as acts of self-advertisement and unethical conduct on the part of the physician. However, printing of sketches, diagrams, picture of human system shall not be treated as unethical.

6.2 Patent and copy rights: A physician may patent surgical instruments, appliances and medicine or copyright applications, methods and procedures. However, it shall be unethical if the benefits of such patents or copyrights are not made available in situations where the interest of large population is involved.

6.3 Running an open shop (dispensing of drugs and appliances by physicians): A physician should not run an open shop for sale of medicine for dispensing prescriptions prescribed by doctors other than himself/herself or for sale of medical or surgical appliances. It is not unethical for a physician to prescribe or supply drugs, remedies or appliances as long as there is no exploitation of the patient. Drugs prescribed by a physician or brought from the market for a patient should explicitly state the proprietary formulae as well as generic name of the drug.

6.4 Rebates and commission:

6.4.1 A physician shall not give, solicit, or receive nor shall he/she offer to give solicit or receive, any gift, gratuity, commission or bonus in consideration of or return for the referring, recommending or procuring of any patient for medical, surgical or other treatment. A physician shall not, directly or indirectly, participate in or be a party to act of division, transference, assignment, subordination, rebating, splitting or refunding of any fee for medical, surgical or other treatment.

6.4.2 Provisions of para 6.4.1 shall apply with equal force to the referring, recommending or procuring by a physician or any person, specimen or material for diagnostic purposes or other study/work. Nothing in this section, however, shall prohibit payment of salaries by a qualified physician to other duly qualified person rendering medical care under his supervision.

6.5 Secret remedies: The prescribing or dispensing by a physician of secret remedial agents of which he/she does not know the composition, or the manufacture or promotion of their use is unethical and as such prohibited. All the drugs prescribed by a physician should always carry a proprietary formula and clear name.

6.6 Human rights: The physician shall not aid or abet torture nor shall he/she be a party to either infliction of mental or physical trauma or concealment of torture inflicted by some other person or agency in clear violation of human rights.

6.7 Euthanasia: Practising euthanasia shall constitute unethical conduct. However, on specific occasion, the question of withdrawing supporting devices to sustain cardio-pulmonary function even after brain death, shall be decided only by a team of doctors and not merely by the treating physician alone. A team of doctors shall declare withdrawal of support system. Such team shall consist of the doctor in charge of the patient, Chief Medical Officer/Medical Officer in-charge of the hospital and a doctor nominated by the in-charge of the hospital from the hospital staff or in accordance with the provisions of the Transplantation of Human Organ Act, 1994.

## 7. MISCONDUCT

The following acts of commission or omission on the part of a physician shall constitute professional misconduct rendering him/her liable for disciplinary action:

7.1 Violation of the regulations: If he/she commits any violation of these regulations.

7.2 If he/she does not maintain the medical records of his/her indoor patients for a period of three years as per regulation 1.3 and refuses to provide the same within 72 hours when the patient or his/her authorized representative makes a request for it as per the regulation 1.3.2.

7.3 If he/she does not display the registration number accorded to him/her by the State Medical Council or the MCI in his/her clinic, prescriptions and certificates, etc., issued by him/her or violates the provisions of regulation 1.4.2.

7.4 Adultery or improper conduct: Abuse of professional position by committing adultery or improper conduct with a patient or by maintaining an improper association with a patient will render a physician liable for disciplinary action as provided under the Indian Medical Council Act, 1956 or the concerned State Medical Council Act.

7.5 Conviction by court of law: Conviction by a court of law for offences involving moral turpitude/criminal acts.

7.6 Sex determination tests: On no account sex determination test shall be undertaken with the intent to terminate the life of a female foetus developing in her mother's womb, unless there are other absolute indications for termination of pregnancy as specified in the Medical Termination of Pregnancy Act, 1971. Any act of termination of pregnancy of normal female foetus amounting to female foeticide shall be regarded as professional misconduct on the part of the physician leading to penal erasure besides rendering him/her liable to criminal proceedings as per the provisions of this Act.

7.7 Signing professional certificates, reports and other documents: Registered medical practitioners are in certain cases bound by law to give, or may from time to time be called upon or requested to give certificates, notification, reports and other documents of similar character signed by them in their professional capacity for subsequent use in the courts or for administrative purposes, etc. Any registered practitioner, who is shown to have signed or given under his/her name and authority any such certificate, notification, report or document of a similar character which is untrue, misleading or improper, is liable to have his name deleted from the register.

7.8 A registered medical practitioner shall not contravene the provisions of the Drugs and Cosmetics Act and regulations made thereunder. Accordingly,

(a) prescribing steroids/psychotropic drugs when there is no absolute medical indication;

(b) selling Schedule 'H' and 'L' drugs and poisons to the public except to his/her patient; in contravention of the above provisions shall constitute gross professional misconduct on the part of the physician.

7.9 Performing or enabling unqualified person to perform an abortion or any illegal operation for which there is no medical, surgical or psychological indication.

7.10 A registered medical practitioner shall not issue certificates of efficiency in modern medicine to unqualified or non-medical person.

*Note:* The foregoing does not restrict the proper training and instruction of bona fide students, midwives, dispensers, surgical attendants, or skilled mechanical and technical assistants and therapy assistants under the personal supervision of physicians.

7.11 A physician should not contribute to the lay press articles and give interviews regarding diseases and treatments which may have the effect of advertising himself/herself or soliciting practices; but is open to write to the lay press under his/her own name on matters of public health, hygienic living or to deliver public lectures, give talks on the radio/TV/internet chat for the same purpose and send announcement of the same to lay press.

7.12 An institution run by a physician for a particular purpose such as a maternity home, nursing home, private hospital, rehabilitation centre or any type of training institution, etc., may be advertised in the lay press, but such advertisements should not contain anything more than the name of the institution, type of patients admitted, type of training and other facilities offered and the fees.

7.13 It is improper for a physician to use an unusually large sign board and write on it anything other than his name, qualifications obtained from a university or a statutory body, titles and name of his speciality, registration number including the name of the State Medical Council under which registered. The same should be the contents of his prescription papers. It is improper to affix a sign board on a chemist's shop or in places where he does not reside or work.

7.14 The registered medical practitioner shall not disclose the secrets of a patient that have been learnt in the exercise of his/her profession except

(i) in a court of law under orders of the Presiding judge;

(ii) in circumstances where there is a serious and identified risk to a specific person and/or community; and

(iii) notifiable diseases.

In case of communicable/notifiable diseases, concerned public health authorities should be informed immediately.

7.15 The registered medical practitioner shall not refuse on religious grounds alone to give assistance in or conduct of sterility, birth control, circumcision and medical termination of pregnancy when there is medical indication, unless the medical practitioner feels himself/herself incompetent to do so.

7.16 Before performing an operation the physician should obtain in writing the consent from the husband or wife, parent or guardian in the case of minor, or the patient himself/herself as the case may be. In an operation which may result in sterility the consent of both husband and wife is needed.

7.17 A registered medical practitioner shall not publish photographs or case reports of his/her patients without their permission, in any medical or other journal in a manner by which their identity could be made out. If the identity is not to be disclosed, the consent is not needed.

7.18 In the case of running of a nursing home by a physician and employing assistants to help him/her, the ultimate responsibility rests on the physician.

7.19 A physician shall not use touts or agents for procuring patients.

7.20 A physician shall not claim to be specialist unless he/she has a special qualification in that branch.

7.21 No act of in-vitro fertilization or artificial insemination shall be undertaken without the informed consent of the female patient and her spouse as well as the donor. Such consent shall be obtained in writing only after the patient is provided, at her own level of comprehension, with sufficient information about the purpose, methods, risks, inconveniences, disappointments of the procedure and possible risks and hazards.

7.22 Research: Clinical drug trials or other research involving patients or volunteers as per the guidelines of ICMR can be undertaken, provided ethical considerations are borne in mind. Violation of existing ICMR guidelines in this regard shall constitute misconduct. Consent taken from the patient for trial of drug or therapy which is not as per the guidelines shall also be construed as misconduct.

7.23 If a physician posted in rural area is found absent on more than two occasions during inspection by the head of the District Health Authority or the Chairman, Zila Parishad, the same shall be construed as a misconduct if it is recommended to the MCI/State Medical Council by the State Government for action under these regulations.

7.24 If a physician posted in a medical college/institution both as teaching faculty or otherwise shall remain in hospital/college during the assigned duty hours. If they are found absent on more than two occasions during this period, the same shall be construed as a misconduct if it is certified by the Principal/Medical Superintendent and forwarded through the State Government to MCI/State Medical Council for action under these regulations.

## 8. PUNISHMENT AND DISCIPLINARY ACTION

8.1 It must be clearly understood that the instances of offences and of professional misconduct which are given above do not constitute and are not intended to constitute a complete list of the infamous acts which calls for disciplinary action, and that by issuing this notice the MCI and/or State Medical Councils are in no way precluded from considering and dealing with any other form of professional misconduct on the part of a registered practitioner. Circumstances may and do arise from time to time in relation to which there may occur questions of professional misconduct which do not come within any of these categories. Every care should be taken that the code is not violated in letter or spirit. In such instances as in all others, the MCI and/or State Medical Councils have to consider and decide upon the facts brought before the MCI and/or State Medical Councils.

8.2 It is made clear that any complaint with regard to professional misconduct can be brought before the appropriate Medical Council for disciplinary action. Upon receipt of any complaint of professional misconduct, the appropriate Medical Council would hold an enquiry and give opportunity to the registered medical practitioner to be heard in person or by pleader. If the medical practitioner is found to be guilty of committing professional misconduct, the appropriate Medical Council may award such punishment as deemed necessary or may direct the removal altogether or for a specified period, from the register of the name of the delinquent registered practitioner. Deletion from the register shall be widely publicized in local press as well as in the publications of different medical associations/societies/bodies.

8.3 In case the punishment of removal from the register is for a limited period, the appropriate Council may also direct that the name so removed shall be restored in the register after the expiry of the period for which the name was ordered to be removed.

8.4 Decision on complaint against delinquent physician shall be taken within a time limit of six months.
8.5 During the pendency of the complaint the appropriate Council may restrain the physician from performing the procedure or practice which is under scrutiny.
8.6 Professional incompetence shall be judged by peer group as per guidelines prescribed by MCI.

## III
## Contemporary Concerns of Women in Medical Ethics

This section will specifically deal with women's respect and equal treatment, informed consent, reproductive issues, technology and womanhood.

The problem of the treatment of women cannot be underestimated when we consider health ethics, equity, human dignity and cultural diversity. In many cultures, even in industrialized countries, women receive less education, less health care and are less involved in decision-making at the family, community or national level than men. In India, generally a woman cannot commit herself to an informed consent unless she takes permission from her husband. In many African countries where AIDS is prevalent, a woman cannot refuse an unsafe sexual relationship with her husband who is infected with AIDS without escaping his punishment. There are examples of cultural issues related to women's health, which exist in spite of the UN convention on elimination of all forms of discrimination against women. They challenge our principles on ethics, equity and human dignity and need more sociological enquiry to empower women through education. We present below some of the areas which are of contemporary concerns to women in the area of medical ethics.

### Women and Equal Medical Care

The traditional interpretation of the physician-patient relationship as a paternalistic one, in which the physician made the decision and the patient submitted to them, has been widely rejected in recent years, both in ethics and law. The Constitution of India provides equality in all respect to men and women, therefore, each individual can make his or her own decision. However, in the patriarchal structure of Indian society, most of the women patients are either unable or unwilling to make decisions about their medical care, thus female patients autonomy is often questioned.

The intimate nature of physician-patient relationship can give rise to sexual attraction. A fundamental rule of traditional medical ethics is that such attraction must be restricted. The oath of Hippocrates includes the following promise: 'whatever houses I may visit, I will come for the benefit of the sick, remaining free of all intentional injustice, of all mischief and in particular of sexual relations with both female and male persons'. In recent years many medical associations have restated this prohibition of sexual relations between physicians and their patients. The reasons for this are as valid today as they were in Hippocrates' time, 2,500 years ago. Women patients are vulnerable and put their trust in physicians to treat them well. They may feel unable to resist sexual advances of physicians for fear that their treatment will be jeopardized. Moreover, the clinical judgement of a physician can be adversely affected by emotional involvement with a patient.

## Women and Informed Consent

Informed consent is one of the central concepts of present-day medical ethics. The right of the patients to make decision about their health has been enshrined in legal and ethical statements in our code of ethics. It states:

> The patient has the right to self-determination, to make free decisions himself/herself. The physician will inform the patient of the consequences of his/her decisions. A mentally competent adult patient has the right to give or withhold consent to any diagnostic procedure or therapy. The patient has the right to the information necessary to make his/her decisions. The patient should understand clearly what is the purpose of any test or treatment, what the result would imply, and what would be the implications of withholding consent.

The 1964 Helsinki Declaration by the World Health Assembly has been revised for a number of times to ensure the safety and rights of human subjects participating as volunteers in drug trials. The Declaration clearly states that the interests of humans should take precedence over the interests of science and society. 'Freely given informed consent' is one of the basic clauses of this code of ethics and should be obtained from each volunteer prior to the clinical trials. The Declaration also lays down that volunteers should be assured of treatment for any injuries resulting from the trials and have the right to withdraw from the research at any point. This is possible if they are informed of the purpose of the research and its risk and potential benefits.

Even the 1994 ICMR document on the clinical trials of contraceptives has very little to contribute in terms of ethical issues. While the mandatory steps for contraceptives approval are delineated, there is no mention of the manner in which trial participants should be recruited, consent should be obtained or long-term follow-up should be done (Srinivasan, 2001). The new ICMR guidelines, on clinical trials, are silent about contraceptive research. They do not address the concerns arising out of their specificities and ensured adequate safeguards. This is essential, firstly, because the bulk of the contraceptive research is targeted towards women – a section of our society that already has lower nutritional levels and poor access to health facilities. Secondly, most of the emerging contraceptive technologies have multi-systemic effects, and require more careful studies in order to ensure their long-term safety vis-à-vis women's health. In addition, of course, is the fact that the impact of such technologies/devices/drugs is not limited only to the health of the research subjects but extends much further and affects the health of future generations (Saheli Women's Resource Centre, 1999). ICMR Code of 2000 on Ethical Guidelines on Biomedical Research Involving Human Subjects has watered down the provisions for mandatory informed consent. In the section on International Collaboration/Assistance in Biomedical Research it talks about the 'best possible nationally available care' instead of international standards thereby bypassing adequate safeguards against exploitation of research volunteers from developing countries. The code thus apparently follows the recent pressures to modify the Helsinki Declaration to make clinical research easier in developing countries. Among the significant changes sought is to permit 'proxy consent' that would eliminate the need for the individual trial participant's consent by obtaining permission from a governmental or non-governmental agency. The second change sought in the Declaration is regarding the standard of care to volunteers: it need not be the 'best-proven care' but rather 'best care available in the country' (Dasgupta, 2004). An anti-cancer drug is not only being widely and wrongly used by doctors to treat infertility in women, but it is also being tested illegally on unaware patients. Letrozole, the drug, has no proven use in curing infertility anywhere in the world. About 400 women were made guinea pig in the Letrozole drug trial for infertility in spite of its side effects (*Hindustan Times*, 21 December 2003).

Abortion is legal in India but only qualified, registered practitioners are allowed to conduct the operation. Since government clinics are absent in many areas, rural practitioners are keen to offer abortion service and make money out of that. At the same time, abortion for women remains social stigma and taboo, the quick and secret services are provided by the rural practitioners make them popular. Dasgupta (2004) found in her study that women who seek quinacrine sterilization (quinacrine is a synthetic anti-malarial chemical used for permanent sterilization which does not require surgery) are neither informed that they are 'volunteers' for a drug trial, nor are they told about the experimental nature of the method and its unknown long-term risks. Doctors simply take advantage of their desperate need for contraception and their ignorance.

The quinacrine sterilization is unethical as the trials for the contraceptives like Net-en and Norplant in India. The only difference is that that the latter trials were legal and conducted by scientific bodies like the ICMR. But, the women who were the 'volunteers' for the Net-en and Norplant trials were recruited through family planning clinics and the experimental nature of the contraceptives and the transaction was hidden from them (Gupta, 2000).

In India, the ideas enshrined in the doctrine of informed consent, though not legally binding yet, continue to percolate into the medical and lay discourse. Many a doubt could be raised about the applicability of such a doctrine to a highly illiterate traditional society such as India, having limited exposure to modern medicine. In such a society the sick person is treated as someone dependent on others, with the family playing a crucial supportive role in the treatment as well as in the patient's interaction with the doctor. The concepts of individual autonomy and freedom of choice in the medical domain, by and large, still remain extrinsic and alien to the Indian thought process. Women patients in India are especially dependent on male relatives when negotiating the external impersonal domain, such as hospital, and dealing with the strangers. It is the family members who take important decisions on their behalf, especially if the decisions are to rest on possessing medical knowledge. During the illness of a woman she is expected to let others assume responsibility for her welfare (Minocha, 2010). Sriram et al. (1991) found that patients felt that the details of the investigations and prognosis need not be always told to them. As for Japan, imposing informed consent on people who do not want medical information and decision-making is ethically wrong and paradoxically paternalistic (Asai, 1996: 91).

## Women and Reproductive Ethical Issues

Many of the most pertinent issues in medical ethics relate to the beginning of human life. These issues are contraception, assisted reproduction, prenatal genetic screening and abortion, etc. The woman has right to control her fertility, including the prevention of unwanted pregnancies. Physicians have to deal with difficult issues such as requests for contraceptives from minors and explaining the risks of different methods. For couples and individuals who cannot conceive naturally, there are various techniques of assisted reproduction, such as artificial insemination, in-vitro fertilization and embryo transfer. Surrogate is another alternative.

Genetic tests are now available for determining whether an embryo or foetus is affected by certain genetic abnormalities and whether it is male or female. Depending on the findings, a decision can be made whether or not to proceed with pregnancy. Since reproduction is so important in a woman's life, therefore, all the decisions related to her reproduction are either decided by the men, or the doctors to whom she is dependent. Physicians need to determine when to offer such tests and how to explain the results to patients. It is also pertinent to note that there is a rampant use of sex-selective technology, which has resulted in skewed sex ratio. Abortion has long been one of most divisive issues in medical ethics, both for physicians and for public authorities.

## Women, Medical Ethics and Emergency

One of the situations experienced by the women in the different health care facilities will explain the ethical dimension during the time of emergency of health care:

> A woman who was supposed to deliver a child was given first aid in a sub-centre and referred to a primary health centre for treatment. The woman was examined at the preliminary level and showed her condition to be serious. Immediate admission for further treatment was recommended. However, she was not admitted in the primary health care facility as there were no vacant beds, and was referred to another district hospital. There too, she was refused admission as there were no vacant beds. Thus, the woman kept on shuttling between different hospitals and at last she went to the private hospital where she had to pay a large amount of money which was difficult for her to pay.

The above incident makes it clear that women are denied admission in the different state health care facilities and that too in the emergency, while the state cannot avoid its obligation just because of no bed vacancy. It has to have an alternative arrangement for the emergency cases.

## Womanhood, Technology and Ethics

Great progress has been achieved in the biomedical field during the last few decades. More is expected in the following decades. Advances in diagnostic imaging and biological testing techniques as well as in medical forecasting based on genetic testing are continuing. The human genome is now deciphered. Advances in surgical and medical cures, organ and tissue plantation, xeno transplantation (i.e., organ transplantation from animals), artificial organs, cloning tissues culture techniques, molecular biology and information technology are reported almost daily. Many ethical issues have been raised and new ethical codes adopted.

The pace of ethical studies needs to be hastened to cope with these rapid advances that may carry serious ethical consequences. As an example, with the advances in foetal surgery, if the mother refuses intervention, because of potential risk to her life, to save her offspring from a fatal or moribund disorder, what are the ethical issues here? The situation is even more complicated if the foetus needing intervention is carried in the womb of a surrogate mother and surrogate mother refuses access through the body while the true mother (who is not carrying the foetus) approves it. Other issue in terms of technology is that the information about the patient which comes under individual genetic privacy right has many openings for research. Should this information about an individual be made public to employer firms, insurance companies, the courts and so on? How can we keep privacy and confidentiality of patient health data that is processed through computers and other machines? Is anonymity a sufficient guarantee for confidentiality? Should we block future epidemic research by blocking all these data? There is thus a need to revise continuously our concepts on ethics.

## IV
## Summary and Conclusions

Ethical analysis of medical and health care policy has a significant implication on the distribution of health care and the role of medical professional in determining the availability of health care services over a period of time. There are some studies done outside India on ethical issues, however, there are very few studies in India which are directly related to medical ethics. Beginning of human history is witnessed by concern for medical ethics in Babylonian, Egyptian, Indian, Chinese and Greek writings. The oath of Hippocrates is considered first such code written in an organized and logical way. The WHO issued the first worldwide ethical code and is modelled after the oath of Hippocrates.

Ethics are concerned with normative questions, reasoning and decisions. Different ethical traditions have developed over a period of time based on western philosophy. Each of these traditions is a product of times in which they were born. Morals are related with practical engagements in particular engagements in a particular local world and cultural specificity. Ethics are globally elaborated abstract articulation over translocal values. However, to talk about universal ethical formulation of justice and equity, without beginning with the local moral condition is useless and irrelevant. Therefore, in the real sense, the distinction has blurred boundaries between moral and ethics and overlaps with its components.

There is a large degree of dispute over the discourse of values and conduct related with the ethics. Aristotle, Kant and Mill represent philosophies of normative moral projects, whereas Beauchamp and Childress and Gillon view that autonomy, beneficence, non-maleficence and justice are binding unless these conflict with another.

India has a long history of medical ethics enunciated in ayurvedic classics around 600 BC and recently in 2002 the Medical Council of India has made the regulations relating to the professional conduct and ethics for registered medical practitioners.

Medical profession is controlled and supervised by the national and state level medical councils. A medical council is empowered to hold an enquiry against doctor suo moto, however, it cannot advance its investigation against unethical practices like organ trade and rebate-commission practices unless the complaint is made.

The codes of medical ethics are for the self-regulation of the medical profession and in turn doctors' duties towards the patient. If the duties are not performed by doctor, his/her right to be a part of the medical profession is questioned.

As stated earlier, the Medical Council Act of 1956 has made some insertions in 2002 relating to the professional conduct, etiquettes and ethics for registered medical practitioners. Every doctor has to sign a declaration of code of conduct. The doctor is expected to uphold the dignity and honour of medical profession and render service to humanity. Every doctor shall maintain medical records of indoor patients under their treatment. The display of registration number given by Medical Council is mandatory. Doctor shall also ensure that there is rational prescription and use of drugs. The personal financial interests of the physician should not conflict with medical interests of the patient. No physician shall refuse treatment to a patient. The doctor should neither exaggerate nor minimize the gravity of patient's condition. Soliciting of patient directly or indirectly by a physician is unethical.

Advances in bio-medical field are putting challenges on ethics in terms of parenthood, genetic ordering, cloning and organ transplantation. Informed consent should be obtained from each volunteer/patient prior to his/her treatment or clinical trial. However, clinical trials are silent about contraceptive research and they do not address the concerns arising out of their specificities and ensure adequate safeguards. The concept of patient autonomy and freedom of choice is silent as most of the patients are illiterate and dependent on others or on family members. The concept of women's autonomy and freedom of choice in the medical domain still remains extrinsic and alien. Women are dependent on men for negotiating the external impersonal domain such as hospital and doctors. Decisions regarding reproduction revolve around the family and women are – not able to decide about her pregnancy and its relevant issues. Providing health care to the women is the state's obligation, however, in number of cases women are refused admission in the different health care facilities. Technology in the field of health care has raised many new emerging ethical concerns regarding the confidentiality of patients, health data, surrogacy, genetic ordering, cloning, etc.

A broad range of issues can be covered under the rubric of ethical issues, however, specific concerns related to the globalization, equity in health, technology and ethics, informed consent, emergency and health care and reproduction are the major concerns of ethics for women.

The ideas enshrined in the doctrine of informed consent, though not legally binding yet, continue to percolate into the medical and lay discourses. The doctrine of informed consent is complicated and needs to be addressed in socio-cultural and other constraints of the society.

Advances in bio-sciences and bio-technology, such as surrogacy, sex selection, genetics, etc., widened the scope of medical ethics. Ethics are the bridge between health policy and values. A nation's health policy is related with the equity and justice to its people in receiving the health care, and thus medical ethics examine the moral validity of it.

There is a need to develop an ethical culture in society. Government should sensitize their own decision-making procedures in the light of ethics. Ethics, equity and respect for humanity must be incorporated in all aspects of health care. Ethics have to be institutionalized wherever these are needed. Independent ethical organizational entities should be established, which can develop new codes of ethics, keeping in view advances and changes in health domain.

## References

Aristotle (1955), *Ethics*, Harmondsworth: Penguin.

Asai, Arushi (1996), 'Barriers to Informed Consent in Japan', *Eubios Journal of Asian and International Bioethics*, Vol. 6, No. 4, pp. 91–93.

Beauchamp, T. and J.E. Childress (1994), *Principles of Biomedical Ethics*, Oxford: Oxford University Press.

British Medical Association (1988), *The Report on the Ethics of Clinical Practice*, UK.

Chapman, Carleton B. (1984), *Physicians, Law and Ethics*, New York: New York University Press.

Code of Ethics Regulations (2002, 2009), Medical Council of India, Amendment Notification, New Delhi, 10 December.

Cohen, L. (1999), 'Where it Hurts: Indian Material for an Ethics of Organ Transplantation', *Daedalus*, Vol. 128, No. 4, pp. 135–66.

Crane, Diana (1975), *The Sanctity of Social Life: Physicians' Treatment of Critically Ill Patients*, New York: Russel Sage.

Daniels, N. et al. (1999), 'Why Justice is Good for Our Health: The Social Determinants of Health Inequalities', *Daedalus*, Vol. 128, No. 4, pp. 215–52.

Dasgupta, Rajashri (2004), 'Quick-fix Medical Ethics: Quinacrine Sterilization and the Ethics of Contraceptive Trials', in Mohan Rao (ed.), *The Unheard Scream: Reproductive Health and Women's Lives in India*, New Delhi: Zubaan, pp. 279–308.

Desai, Prakash N. (1988), 'Medical Ethics in India', *The Journal of Medicine and Philosophy*, Vol. 13, No. 3, pp. 231–55.

Desai, Mihir and Dipti Chand (2007), 'Right to Emergency Health Care', in Mihir Desai and Kamayani Bali Mahabal (eds), *Health Care Case Law in India: A Reader*, Mumbai: Centre for Enquiry into Health and Allied Themes (CEHAT).

Farmer, P. (1999), *Infections and Inequalities*, Berkeley: University of California Press.

Fox, Renee C. (1974), 'Ethical and Existential Developments in Contemporaneous American Medicine: Their Implications for Culture and Society', *Milbank Memorial Fund Quarterly*, Vol. 52, pp. 445–83.

Freidson, Eliot (1970), *Professional Dominance: The Social Structure of Medical Care*, New Jersey: Transaction Publishers.

Gillon, R. (1994), 'Medical Ethics: Four Principles Plus Attention to Scope', *British Medical Journal*, Vol. 309, Fall, pp. 184–88.

Gottlieb, N., J. Burdine and K. McLeroy (eds) (1987), 'Ethical Dilemmas in Health Promotion', *Health Education Quarterly*, Vol. 14, Spring, pp. 1–109.

Gupta, Jyotsna Agnihotri (2000), *New Reproductive Technologies: Women's Health and Autonomy: Freedom or Dependency?*, New Delhi: Sage Publications.

*Hindustan Times* (2003), 21 December.

Jayshri, K. (2011), 'Organ Transplantation: Legal, Social and Ethical Issues', 5 April, *www.legalserviceindia.com*.

Kleinman, Arthur (2004), 'Ethics and Experience: An Anthropological Approach to Health Equity', in Sudhir Anand, Fabienne Peter and Amartya Sen (eds), *Public Health, Ethics and Equity*, New York: Oxford University Press.

Lustig, B.A. et al. (1993), *Bioethics Yearbook*, Vol. 2, Dordrecht: Kluwer Academic Publishing.

Mathiharan, Karunakaran (2011), 'Ethical and Legal Issues in Organ Transplantation: Indian Scenario', *Medicine, Science and Law*, Vol. 51, No. 3, July, pp. 134–40.

Mechanic, David (1979), *Future Issues in Health Care: Social Policy and the Rationing of Medical Services*, New York: Free Press.

——. (ed.) (1983), *Handbook of Health, Health Care and the Health Professors*, New York: Free Press.

Mechanic, David and L.H. Aiken (1986), *Application of Social Science to Clinical Medicine and Health Policy*, New Brunswick, NJ: Rutgers University Press.

Mill, J.S. (1962), *Utilitarianism and Other Writings*, London: Fontana.

Minocha, Anita (2010), 'Informed Consent in Medical Practice', in B.S. Baviskar and Tulsi Patel (eds), *Understanding Indian Society: Past and Present*, New Delhi: Orient Blackswan.

Nagla, Madhu (1997), *Sociology of Medical Profession*, Jaipur: Rawat Publications.

Pandya, Sunil (2000), 'History of Medical Ethics in India', *Eubios Journal of Asian and International Bioethics*, Vol. 10, pp. 40–44.

Saheli Women's Resource Centre (1999), *The Consultative Document on Ethical Guidelines on Biomedical Research Involving Human Trials: A Critique and Some Recommendations*, September.

Simmons, R. and M. Di Canio (1979), 'Biology, Technology and Health', in H. Freeman, S. Levine and L. Reeder (eds), *Handbook of Medical Sociology*, Englewood Cliffs, NJ: Prentice-Hall, pp. 150–73.

Srinivasan, Sandhya (2001), 'Discussion on Biomedical Research on Human in India: A Short Review', paper presented at the Workshop on Research Ethics in South Asia, Thiruvananthapuram, Achutha Menon Centre for Health Science Studies.

Sriram, T.G. et al. (1991), 'Informed Consent: A Study of Experiences and Opinion of Utilizers of Health Services from India', *Social Science and Medicine*, Vol. 32, No. 12, pp. 1389–92.

Stacey, Margaret (1985), 'Medical Ethics and Medical Practice: A Social Science View', *Journal of Medicine Ethics*, Vol. 11, pp. 14–18.

Susser, M., W. Watson and K. Hopper (1985), *Sociology in Medicine*, New York: Oxford University Press.

*The Times of India* (2012), 'Shaming the Hippocratic Oath', 4 June.

Vashistha, Vipin M. (2010), 'MCIs New Code of Ethics for Medical Professionals: An Exercise in Vain or a Welcome Move', *Indian Paediatrics*, Vol. 47, 17 April, pp. 329–30.

Wig, K.L. (1985), 'Medical and Ethical Issues of Population: Reflection of a Physician', delivered a keynote address in the Plenary Session on 23 February in World Congress of Law and Medicine, New Delhi.

# 7 Girl Child Health in India

To be born and brought up in healthy conditions is the right of every child. In 1987 the SAARC conference on South Asian Children made an urgent call for improvement of the mother-child life cycle starting with the girl child. This desire took a concrete form by the decision taken at SAARC summit held in 1988 to declare 1990 as the *Year of the Girl Child*.

In India, inhumane and deliberate neglect of the girl child has the support of religious sanctions and traditional practices and family support. The socio-cultural variables influence the rearing of the girl child right from the birth and restrict her role in the primary groups such as family and friends. The girl child at home shares the responsibilities of the household, i.e., looking after her siblings, grazing cattle, sweeping, cleaning, cooking, washing, collecting fodder, fuel, fetching water, etc. She contributes substantially to the sustenance and growth of the household economy but her condition is neither acknowledged by the elders nor compensated.

In most populations, female mortality rates are lower than those for males at all ages (Hill and Upchurch, 1995: 129), apparently both because of male's higher degree of biologically-based susceptibility to disease and because of a higher prevalence of poor health habits and risky behaviour, especially among adolescents and adult men (Waldron, 1986). However, in many parts of South Asia with strong son preference attitudes, the situation is reversed with higher mortality for females particularly during the second half of the first year and childhood (Arnold, 1997; D'Souza and Chen,

1980; Meegama, 1980). The evidence of an excess of female deaths in childhood is usually interpreted as the result of parental discrimination against daughters in the allocation of food (Behram, 1988; Chen et al., 1981) and health care (Rahaman et al., 1982), neglect or even abuse of girls (Miller, 1981) and relative medical and nutritional neglect of the girl child (Das Gupta, 1987; Basu, 1989) within the household. It has also been postulated that where behaviour can be sufficiently powerful to influence outcome, there is consistent discrimination against female children in comparison to male children (Chen et al., 1981: 66).

There is a growing body of literature which suggests that girls in India are discriminated against in the provision of health care but are not neglected in nutritional allocations. For example, in studies of six Deccan villages surveyed by ICRISAT, Walker and Ryan (1990) find that more boys than girls of pre-school (1–6) and school-age (7–12) were poorly nourished on a standard weight-for-age. In two studies of North and South Indian residents of a Delhi slum, Basu (1989, 1993) finds that despite supposed greater discrimination against girls in northern India, there was a higher incidence of severe malnutrition among boys in North Indian sample. The converse was true in the South Indian sample. Indeed, North Indian girls had a slightly better diet than their brothers in the case of some choice of foods such as fruit and eggs, although they fared a little worse in milk consumption. Numerous other studies (e.g., Chaudhury, 1987; Gopalan, 1987; Nutritional Foundation of India, 1988) suggest that nutritional imbalances are not a major part of gender inequalities in the region.

On the other hand, Singh, Gordon and Wyon (1962) find that girls in rural Punjab receive less and worse medical care than boys in the treatment of fatal illness. Aziz (1977) finds that, of boys and girls who perish of illness in Bangladesh girls are less likely to receive medical care. Chen, Huq and D'Souza (1981) find that, despite free treatment of diarrhoeal disease in a *thana* (sub-district administrative unit in Bangladesh and equal incidence of diarrhoea among boys and girls, boys are more likely to be brought to the treatment centre. Summary of data from the NFHS (Kurz and Johnson-Welch, 1997) also suggests that boys are more likely to be immunized and receive health care at a medical facility.

The strong preference for sons over daughters and resulting discrimination against daughters in India is well known, though the preference is not uniformly observed across different regions of the country. India exhibits wide variations in the degree of son's preference, with stronger son preference found in northern India than in the south (Dyson and Moore, 1983). A review of literature on this topic indicates that while the existing studies in India document the existence of sex bias, detailed state level explorations into the extent, pattern and nature of gender disparity in various possible parameters of discrimination have not been undertaken. Most research of this type has been concentrated on the Punjab state of India (Das Gupta, 1987).

This paper deals with Haryana state of North India. It examines patterns of gender disparities for children in health outcomes, including disease incidence, use of preventive and curative health care services and nutrition. The focus on health outcomes for children is mainly for the reason that these outcomes, such as child morbidity, are relatively less influenced by choices of the children themselves and potentially more indicative of differential treatment by their parents (and other adults) and hence may indicate more clearly one particular source of gender disparity. Specifically it addresses the following questions: Are boys more likely to have complete vaccination coverage than girls? Are girls more likely to suffer from diarrhoea? Are boys more likely to receive care for an episode of diarrhoea, and are they more likely to receive 'better' care than girls? Are girls more likely to be malnourished than boys? If so, does the extent of pro-male bias depend on various socio-economic and demographic factors?

Knowledge of levels and patterns of sex differentials in ill-health, malnutrition and treatment is important for policy makers and programme mangers to understand in order to (i) ensure equitable access to service utilization, and (ii) avoid any adverse impact on a preference in a population. For example, a high level of son preference in countries with low level of fertility has resulted in a skewed sex ratio at birth because the women have access to methods of identifying the sex of foetuses and to induced abortions (Park and Cho, 1995). A skewed sex ratio, in turn, has worrisome implications for future population structure, the marriage and labour market, and personality development. In this regard, population policy needs to pay special attention to the possible consequences of high son preference that go beyond the retardation of fertility decline. This is particularly important in states like Haryana where the practice of sex-selective abortion is most widespread (Das Gupta and Mari Bhat, 1997: 312).

Sex discrimination in nutrition has implications for reproductive health. Some women face difficulties in carrying a pregnancy successfully to completion because of childhood discrimination (Royston and Armstrong, 1989). Failure to nourish girl children can limit their capacity for healthy motherhood through, for example, stunting and a small pelvis, while a reluctance to provide medical care may compound these problems (WHO, 1998). If a pregnancy goes wrong, lack of obstetric care may be fatal and millions of women continue to face such risks every year (Thaddeus and Maine, 1991; Royston and Armstrong, 1989).

Haryana provides an ideal situation for exploring gender disparity in child health. It is a fairly well-developed state with third highest per capita income in India (Government of India, 2001). It is also a state which has shown strong evidence of son preference (see Table 1). It has the most unbalanced child sex ratio in India (Registrar General of India, 2001), which is a grim indicator of the persistence and severity of discrimination against girls and women. Of the ten districts with lowest child sex ratio in India, four are in Haryana (Registrar General of India, 1991). UNICEF argued that 'female foeticide' is reported to be a cause for adverse sex ratio in some Indian districts in the 1991 Census (UNICEF, 1995).

The pattern of sex differentials in mortality by age provides evidence of differential treatment of male and female children leading to higher mortality risks for females. The mortality rate for girls is considerably higher than for boys in every age group below five years (see Table 2). The ratio of female to male mortality rates ranges from a low of 1.1 in the case of neonatal mortality[1] to a high of 2.1 in the case of child mortality (age 1.4 years) (IIPS, 2001). According to a World Bank study (Filmer et al., 1998), the ratio of female to male child mortality in Haryana is worse than in any country in the world. This is a state where technical means to identify sex through amniocentesis and ultrasound have been used to accommodate the widespread preference for sons (George and Dahiya, 1998).

**Table 1** ***Selected indicators of son preference, Haryana and India, 1992–93 and 1998–99***

| *Indicators* | *Haryana* | | *India* | |
|---|---|---|---|---|
| | *1992–93* | *1998–99* | *1992–93* | *1998–99* |
| Ratio ideal number sons/daughters | 1.6 | 1.6 | 1.5 | 1.4 |
| Proportion fully vaccinated (boys/girls) | 1.13 | 0.99 | 1.08 | 1.05 |
| Median duration breastfeeding (boys/girls) | 1.24 | 1.10 | 1.07 | |
| Prevalence of diarrhoea (boys/girls) | 0.94 | 0.85 | 1.05 | 1.02 |
| Proportion taken to a health facility or provider (boys/girls) | 1.02 | 1.03 | 1.06 | 1.04 |
| Proportion undernourished (girls/boys) | 1.19 | 1.20 | 1.00 | 1.08 |
| Proportion stunted (girls/boys) | 1.12 | 1.12 | 0.99 | 1.06 |
| Child mortality (ages 1–4 (female/male) | 2.34 | 2.19 | 1.42 | 1.47 |
| Excess female child mortality (%) | 135 | 119 | 43 | 47 |

*Source:* National Family and Health Survey, Haryana and India, 1992–93 and 1998–99.

**Table 2** ***Neonatal, post-neonatal, child and under-five mortality by sex of the child in Haryana State, 1998–99***

| *Age Group* | *Total* | *Male* | *Female* | *Ratio Female/ Male* |
|---|---|---|---|---|
| Neonatal mortality | 34.0 | 32.2 | 36.0 | 1.11 |
| Postneonatal mortality | 25.0 | 20.6 | 30.0 | 1.45 |
| Infant mortality | 59.0 | 52.9 | 66.0 | 1.24 |
| Child mortality | 21.4 | 13.8 | 30.2 | 2.18 |
| Under-five mortality | 79.1 | 66.0 | 94.2 | 1.42 |

*Notes:* Neonatal mortality: the probability of dying in the first month of life;
Postneonatal mortality: the difference between infant and neonatal mortality
Infant mortality: the probability of dying before the first birthday;
Child mortality: the probability of dying between the first and fifth birthday;
Under-five mortality: the probability of dying before the fifth birthday.

*Source:* IIPS (2001).

The female life expectancy in Haryana is 1.4 years less than for males (63.4 years for males and 62 for females) (IIPS, 1995). The birth rate is high (TFR is 4 compared to 3.6 for India as a whole). Women with sons in Haryana are more likely to want to stop having children and use contraception than women with daughters. By this measure, among all the states of India, son preference is strongest in Haryana (Mutharayappa et al., 1997). Despite exhibiting strong preference, there has been little exploration of the nature of gender disparity in child health in Haryana.

## Methods and Data Used

The data for this paper are mainly drawn from the Second National Family and Health Survey (NFHS-2), undertaken in 1998–99. But, the qualitative results are supported by qualitative information obtained during a field survey conducted between December 2000 and February 2001. The qualitative data comprised of in-depth interviews with key functionaries, informal interviews with women and participant observation. The NFHS-2 (Haryana) covered a representative sample of more than 90,000 ever-married women aged 15–49. In Haryana, NFHS-2 collected information from 2,908 eligible women. The analyses for this paper are based on data from a sub-sample of 994 children born to eligible women in the three years preceding the surveys and who were alive at the time of survey. The NFHS-2 provides high-quality, up-to-date information on all the key variables required for the analysis. It has collected extensive information on child health indicators such as immunization coverage, prevalence and treatment of diarrhoea among children, and anthropometric indicators of nutritional status for children born three years preceding the survey – all of which can be examined by sex of child.

One important feature of this study is the small number of cases on which the analyses are based. The present study focuses on child health among alive children below three years of age in Haryana state. Only 994 cases met the criteria. This limitation might have an effect on the analysis, in particular, the small number of cases will limit the statistical methods to be used. This is particularly important in the analyses of the morbidity data on the occurrence and treatment of diarrhoea when only 136 children were reported as having diarrhoea during the two weeks preceding the survey. Even with a short recall period of two weeks, and extensive training of interviewers, the chances of underreporting or misreporting cannot be discounted. Overreporting, on the other hand, is unlikely, so that measures have an inherent negative bias. In addition, since all children who met the criteria were included in the analyses, some characteristics of women and their husbands may be duplicated if they had more than one child. However, the number of children who fall in such groups is quite small, and thus will not have a significant effect on variables under study.

## Health Status of Children

It is expressed in terms of immunization status, prevalence of diarrhoea and its treatment, anthropometrics among children.

Table 3 presents information about the sample that was used in this analysis and summarizes some of its characteristics. Of the mothers in the sample, around 50 per cent have received no education, compared with 23 per cent of the fathers. This finding is congruent with the lower levels of female literacy in Haryana. It also indicates that 77 per cent of the children live in rural areas, 53 per cent have access to piped water, flush or pit toilet, 42 per cent own a television, refrigerator or motorcycle, 60 per cent watch television every week and 30 per cent listen to radio every week.

**Table 3** ***Percentage of children under age three years according to selected demographic and socio-economic characteristics, Haryana, 1998–99***

| *Variables* | *Percentage* | *Number of Children* |
|---|---|---|
| **Bio-maternal characteristics** | | |
| Mother's age at birth of child (years) | | |
| <19 | 10.2 | 101 |
| 20–29 | 74.2 | 740 |
| 30+ | 15.4 | 153 |
| Preceding birth interval | | |
| First birth/>_24 months or more | 18.3 | 182 |
| <24 months | 81.7 | 812 |
| **Child's characteristics** | | |
| Sex of the child | | |
| Male | 55.2 | 549 |
| Female | 44.8 | 445 |
| Age of the child in months | | |
| <6 | 19.4 | 193 |
| 6–11 | 14.1 | 140 |
| 12–23 | 33.6 | 334 |
| 24–35 | 32.9 | 327 |

*Cont'd...*

...*Cont'd*

| | | |
|---|---|---|
| Birth order | | |
| 1 | 29.2 | 290 |
| 2–3 | 46.4 | 461 |
| 4+ | 24.4 | 243 |
| **Socio-economic characteristics** | | |
| Education level of mother | | |
| Illiterate | 49.1 | 488 |
| Literate | 50.9 | 506 |
| Education level of father | | |
| Illiterate | 23.0 | 229 |
| Literate | 77.0 | 765 |
| Mother's current work status | | |
| Not employed | 93.3 | 927 |
| Employed | 6.7 | 67 |
| Caste/Tribe | | |
| Scheduled Caste | 24.7 | 246 |
| Non-Scheduled Caste | 75.3 | 748 |
| Religion | | |
| Hindu | 86.1 | 856 |
| Non-Hindu | 13.9 | 138 |
| Area of residence | | |
| Urban | 23.3 | 232 |
| Rural | 76.7 | 762 |
| Access to amenities (piped water, flush or pit toilet) | | |
| None | 46.9 | 466 |
| One/both | 53.1 | 528 |
| Ownership of television or refrigerator or motorcycle | | |
| None | 41.6 | 414 |
| One/two/all three | 58.4 | 580 |
| Watch television every week | | |
| No | 40.6 | 404 |
| Yes | 59.4 | 590 |
| Listen to radio every week | | |
| No | 69.8 | 694 |
| Yes | 30.2 | 300 |
| Total | 100 | 994 |

*Source:* National Family and Health Survey, Haryana (1998–99).

The first step in the analysis is to consider immunization coverage among the sub-sample of children aged 12–35 months. Based on information obtained from a cared or reported by the mother ('either source'), 65.5 per cent of children aged 12–35 months are fully vaccinated, and only 8 per cent have not received any vaccination. Coverage for each vaccination is much higher than the percentage of fully vaccinated (see Table 4). Although DPT and polio vaccination are given at the same time as part of routine immunization, the coverage rates are slightly higher for polio than for DPT, which may be because of Pulse Polio[2] campaigns. The overall figures for immunization coverage suggest that girls are slightly more likely to be fully vaccinated than boys (66% versus 65%). However, girls are slightly less likely to have received each of the individual vaccinations except measles. Mothers showed vaccination card for 26 per cent of boys and 22 per cent of girls.[3]

**Table 4** ***Percentage of children aged 12–35 months by source of information and specific vaccination, according to the sex of the child, Haryana, 1998–99***

| *Vaccination Source* | *Percentage Vaccinated* | | |
|---|---|---|---|
| | *Boys* | *Girls* | *Girls/Boys* |
| Has vaccination card | 56.2 | 59.8 | 1.06 |
| Percentage fully vaccinated | 65.1 | 66.0 | 1.01 |
| Percentage ever vaccinated | 92.4 | 91.4 | 0.98 |
| Vaccines | | | |
| BCG | 88.9 | 89.3 | 1.00 |
| DPT-1 | 90.8 | 90.4 | 0.99 |
| DPT-2 | 88.1 | 86.3 | 0.97 |
| DPT-3 | 76.2 | 75.9 | 0.99 |
| Polio-1 | 92.2 | 91.4 | 0.99 |
| Polio-2 | 90.3 | 88.0 | 0.97 |
| Polio-3 | 75.1 | 74.6 | 0.99 |
| Measles | 77.0 | 78.1 | 1.01 |
| Total | 370 | 291 | 661 |

*Source:* National Family and Health Survey, Haryana (1998–99).

The next set of questions relates to the occurrence of diarrhoea and the treatment that is provided to children who have diarrhoea. Table 5 shows that 14 per cent of children under age three suffered from diarrhoea in the two-week period before the interview. Among children under age three, boys (13%) are somewhat less likely to have suffered from diarrhoea than girls (15%). This table also shows the percentage of boys and girls under age three with diarrhoea during the two weeks preceding the survey, who were and were not treated for diarrhoea, and where they were treated. For 93 per cent of children in Haryana who suffered from diarrhoea during the two weeks preceding the survey, medical advice or treatment was sought from a health facility or provider (a much higher percentage than the national level of 63%). Seven per cent of children with diarrhoea did not receive any treatment at all.

Table 5 also indicates that the proportion of children not treated is slightly higher among girls than among boys (7.6%, compared with 5.8%), and the proportion of children who are taken to a health facility is slightly higher among boys than girls (94.2%, compared with 92.4%). But, the proportion of children taken to a private health facility is also slightly higher for girls than for boys (75.8%, compared with 73.9%).

**Table 5** ***Percentage of children under age three who were ill with diarrhoea during the two weeks preceding the survey and who were and were not treated for diarrhoea, by where they were treated, according to the sex of the child, Haryana, 1998–99***

| *Children with diarrhoea where treated* | *Boys* | *Girls* | *Girls/Boys* |
|---|---|---|---|
| With diarrhoea | 12.9 | 15.11 | 1.17 |
| Not treated | 5.8 | 7.6 | 1.31 |
| Private health facility | 73.9 | 75.8 | 1.02 |
| Public health facility | 13.0 | 12.1 | 0.93 |
| Both private and public | 7.2 | 4.5 | 0.62 |
| Total children | 542 | 437 | 979 |

*Source:* National Family and Health Survey, Haryana (1998–99).

The last set of questions relates to the nutritional status of boys and girls. Table 6 shows nutritional status of children in Haryana as calculated according to 'weight-for-age' and 'height-for-age' measures.[4] Discrimination against girls in Haryana is particularly pronounced in the nutritional status of children as depicted by these two nutritional indices. Undernutrition is more common among female children than male children. For instance, 38 per cent of female children, compared to 32 per cent of male children, are underweight and 53 per cent of female children compared to 48 per cent of male children are stunted.

**Table 6** ***Percentage of children under age three years classified as undernourished on three anthropometric indices of nutritional status, according to the sex of the child, Haryana, 1998–99***

| *Anthropometric indices* | *Boys* | *Girls* | *Girls/Boys* |
|---|---|---|---|
| Weight-for-age (underweight) | | | |
| Percentage below-2SD[1] | 31.8 | 38.0 | 1.19 |
| Height for age (stunted) | | | |
| Percentage below 2SD[1] | 47.6 | 53.2 | 1.11 |
| Both underweight and stunted | | | |
| Percentage below – SD[1] | 27.3 | 31.1 | 1.13 |
| Total children | 487 | 389 | 876 |

*Note:* Each index is expressed in Standard Deviation (SD) units from the median of the International Reference Population.
[1]Includes children who are below – 3SD from the International Reference Population median.

*Source:* National Family and Health Survey, Haryana (1998–99).

## Efforts by Haryana Government to Check Foeticide

Despite introducing new schemes and incentives to check female foeticide by the state government in the state, it has hit a new road block with the deteriorating sex ratio in urban cities like Gurgaon. So, to encourage the urban women, the government has made a series of efforts including offering work-time options for women employees in government offices. Under this, they can work half day and take much of salary for a maximum of five years. Haryana would be the first state to initiate such initiative. The government is also working out modalities for loans for higher studies for girls with banks. The maximum interest rate for such loan would not be above 5 per cent. Urban educated would get the maximum benefit of this scheme and the maximum amount could go up to ₹ 20 lakh. Government has also announced that the persons informing the health department of any foeticide in the state would be rewarded with ₹ 5,000. To fight this tragedy, 300 delivery huts have already been in operation in the state (*The Times of India*, 5 January 2007, New Delhi).

## Notes

1. A slightly higher neonatal mortality rate for girls than for boys (12% higher) is unexpected, because neonatal mortality (which largely reflects mortality due to congenital conditions) tends to be higher for boys than for girls in most populations. Neonatal mortality was higher for boys than for girls in NFHS-1 (IIPS, 1995).
2. These results show that there has been considerable improvement in full vaccination coverage in Haryana since NFHS-1, when the proportion of children fully vaccinated was 54 per cent. The proportion of children who did not receive any vaccination declined substantially, from 18 per cent in NFHS-1 to 8 per cent in NFHS-2. The coverage of each specific vaccination has also improved considerably since NFHS-1, suggesting that many more children were brought into the programme in the six years between the two surveys.
3. In NFHS-1, vaccination coverage was higher for boys than for girls and vaccination cards were shown for a higher proportion of boys than of girls.
4. The two nutritional status indices provide somewhat different information about nutritional status of children. The height for age index measures linear growth retardation among children. Children who are more than two standard deviations below the median of the reference population in terms of height-for-age are considered short for their age or stunted. The percentage in this category indicates the prevalence of chronic undernutrition which often leads to chronic or recurrent diarrhea. Stunting is typically associated with inadequate food intake resulting from poor feeding practices or from the lack of sufficient food, as well as the existence of adverse environmental conditions for an extended period of time. Height-for-age, therefore, is a measure of the long-term effects of undernutrition. Weight-for-age is a composite measure which takes into account both chronic and acute undernutrition. Children who are more than two standard deviations below the reference median on this index are considered underweight.

## References

Arnold, F. (1997), 'Gender Preferences for Children: Findings from the Demographic and Health Surveys', paper presented for the 23rd General Population Conference of the International Union for the Scientific Study of Population (IUSSP), Beijing, 11–17 October.

Arnold, F., M.K. Choe and T.K. Roy (1998), 'Son Preference, the Family Building Process, and Child Mortality in India', *Population Studies*, Vol. 52, No. 2, pp. 301–15.

Aziz, K.M.A. (1977), 'Present Trends in Medical Consultations Prior to Death in Rural Bangladesh', *Bangladesh Medical Journal*, Vol. 6.

Basu, A.M. (1989), 'Is Discrimination in Food Really Necessary for Explaining Sex Differences in Childhood Mortality?', *Population Studies*, Vol. 43, No. 2, pp. 193–210.

Basu, A.M. (1993), 'How Pervasive are Sex Differentials in Childhood Nutritional Levels in South Asia?', *Social Biology*, Vol. 40, Nos 1–2, pp. 25–37.

Black, R.E. (1984), 'Diarrheal Diseases and Child Morbidity and Mortality', in W.H. Mosley and L.C. Chen (eds), *Child Survival Strategies for Research Population and Development Review*, A Supplement to Vol. 10, pp. 141–61.

Black, R.E., K.H. Brown and S. Becker (1984), 'Malnutrition is a Determining Factor in Diarrheal Duration, but Not Incidence among Young Children in a Longitudinal Study in Rural Bangladesh', *American Journal of Clinical Nutrition*, Vol. 39, pp. 82–94.

Behrman, J.R. (1988), 'Intrahousehold Allocation of Nutrients in Rural India: Are Boys Favoured? Do Parents Exhibit Inequality Aversion?', Oxford Economic Papers, Vol. 40, No. 1, pp. 32–54.

Briscoe, J.L.S.A., J.S. Akin, D.K. Guilkey, B.M. Popkin, R.E. Black and W. Flieger (1991), 'Underlying and Proximate Determinants of Child Health: The Cebu Longitudinal Health and Nutrition Study', *American Journal of Epidemiology*, Vol. 133, No. 2, pp. 185–201.

Caldwell, J.C. (1979), 'Education as a Factor in Mortality Decline: An Examination of Nigerian Data', *Population Studies*, Vol. 23, No. 2, pp. 395–413.

Chaudhury, R.H. (1987), 'Dietary Adequacy and Sex Bias: Preschool Children in Rural Bangladesh', *Social Action*, Vol. 31.

Chen, L.C., E. Huq and S. D'Souza (1981), 'Sex Bias in the Family Allocation of Food and Health Care in Rural Bangladesh', *Population and Development Review*, Vol. 7, No. 1, pp. 55–70.

Das Gupta, M. (1987), 'Selective Discrimination against Female Children in Rural Punjab, India', *Population and Development Review*, Vol. 13, No. 1, pp. 77–100.

Das Gupta, M. and P.N. Mari Bhat (1997), 'Fertility Decline and Increased Manifestation of Sex Bias in India', *Population Studies*, Vol. 51, No. 3, pp. 307–15.

D'Souza, S. and L.C. Chen (1980), 'Sex Differentials in Mortality in Rural Bangladesh', *Population and Development Review*, Vol. 6, No. 2, pp. 257–70.

Dyson, T. and M. Moore (1983), 'On Kinship Structure, Female Autonomy, and Demographic Balance', *Population and Development Review*, Vol. 9, No. 1, pp. 35–60.

Filmer, D., E.M. King and L. Pritchett (1998), 'Gender Disparity in South Asia: Comparisons between and within Countries', World Bank Working Paper No. 1867.

George, S.M. and R.S. Dahiya (1998), 'Female Foeticide in Rural Haryana', *Economic and Political Weekly*, Vol. 33, No. 32, 8 August, pp. 2191–98.

Gopalan, C. (1987), 'Gender Bias in Health and Nutrition Care', *Nutrition Foundation of India Bulletin 8*.

Government of India (1998), *Annual Report 1997–98*, Ministry of Health and Family Welfare, New Delhi.

——. (2001), *Economic Survey*, Central Statistical Organisation, New Delhi.

Hill, K. and D.M. Upchurch (1995), 'Gender Differences in Child Health: Evidence from the Demographic and Health Surveys', *Population and Development Review*, Vol. 21, No. 1, pp. 127–51.

International Institute for Population Sciences (IIPS) (1995), *National Family Health Survey, Haryana, 1992–93*, Bombay.

——. (2001), *National Family Health Survey, Haryana, 1998–99*, Bombay.

Kurz, K.M. and C. Johnson-Welch (1997), 'Gender Bias in Health Care among Children 0–5 Years: Opportunities for Child Survival Programmes', BASICS Review Paper, International Center for Research on Women.

Meegama, S.A. (1980), 'Socio-economic Determinants of Infant and Child Mortality in Sri Lanka: An Analysis of Post-war Experience', *WFS Scientific Reports*, No. 8, London: World Fertility Survey.

Miller, B.D. (1981), *The Endangered Sex: Neglect of Female Children in Rural North India*, Ithaca, NY: Cornell University Press.

Mutharayappa, R., M.K. Choe, F. Arnold and T.K. Roy (1997), 'Son Preference and its Effect on Fertility in India', *National Family Health Survey Subject Reports*, No. 3, International Institute for Population Sciences, Mumbai, India and East-West Center, Programme on Population, Honolulu, Hawaii, USA.

Nutritional Foundation of India (1988), 'Profile of Undernutrition and Underdevelopment: Studies of Poor Communities in Seven Regions of the Country', *NFI Scientific Report*, No. 8, Delhi.

Park, C.B. and N.H. Cho (1995), 'Consequences of Son Preference in Low Fertility Countries in East Asia: Rising Imbalance of Sex Ratio at Birth', *Population and Development Review*, Vol. 21, pp. 59–84.

Rahaman, M.M., K.M.S. Aziz, M.H. Munshi, Y. Patwani and M. Rahman (1982), 'A Diarrhea Clinic in Rural Bangladesh: Influence of Distance, Age, and Sex on Attendance and Diarrhea Mortality', *American Journal of Public Health*, Vol. 72, p. 1124.

Registrar General of India (1991), Census of India, Primary Census Abstract, General Population, Series I-India, Part II-B (i).

——. (2001), Census of India 2001, Provisional Population Totals, Series 1, Paper 1 of 2001, Office of Registrar General and Census Commissioner, New Delhi.

Royston, E. and S. Armstrong (1989), *Preventing Maternal Deaths*, Geneva: World Health Organisation.

Schutz, P.T. (1984), 'Studying the Impact of Household Economic and Community Variables on Child Mortality', in W.H. Mosley and L.C. Chen (eds), *Population and Development Review, Supplement to Vol. 10, Child Survival: Strategies for Research*, New York: Cambridge University Press.

Singh, S.J.E. Gordon and J.B. Wyon (1962), 'Medical Care in Fatal Illness of a Rural Punjab Population: Some Social, Biological and Cultural Factors and their Ecological Implications', *Indian Journal of Medical Research*, Vol. 50, November.

Thaddeus, S. and D. Maine (1991), *Too Far to Walk: Maternal Mortality in Context*, New York: Centre for Population and Family Health, Faculty of Medicine, Columbia University.

Tomkins, A. and F. Watson (1989), 'Malnutrition and Infection', in A. Tomkins and F. Watson (eds), *Malnutrition and Infection: A Review*, ACC/SCN State-of-the-Art Series, Nutrition Policy Discussion Paper No. 5, UN Administrative Committee on Coordination-Subcommittee on Nutrition.

Trehan, M. and S. Sethi (1980), 'A Time for Reckoning', *India Today*, 1–15 August, pp. 34–37.

UNICEF (1995), *The State of the World Children*, Oxford: Oxford University Press.

Waldron, I. (1986), 'What Do We Know About Causes of Sex Differences in Mortality? A Review of the Literature', *Population Bulletin of United Nations*, Vol. 18, pp. 59–76.

Walker, T.S. and J.G. Ryan (1990), *Village and Household Economies in India's Semi-Arid Tropics*, Baltimore, MD: Johns Hopkins University Press.

World Health Organisation (WHO) (1998), *Gender and Health: Technical Paper*, Women's Health and Development, Geneva.

# 8 Obstetrical Care Decisions Among Village Women

## The Case of Haryana

In rural areas, the government delivers reproductive and other health services through its network of Primary Health Centres (PHCs), sub-centres, and other health facilities. In addition, pregnant women and children can obtain services from private maternity homes, hospitals, private practitioners, and in some cases, non-governmental organizations (NGOs). In urban areas reproductive health services are available mainly through government or municipal hospitals, private hospitals and nursing homes. In rural areas, a female paramedical worker, called an auxiliary nurse midwife (ANM), is posted at a sub-centre to provide basic maternal health, child health, and family welfare services to women and children either in their homes or in the health clinic. Her work is overseen by a leady health visitor (LHV) posted at the PHC. With regard to safe motherhood, the ANM is responsible for registering pregnant women, motivating them to obtain antenatal and postnatal care, assessing their health throughout pregnancy and in the postpartum period, and referring women with high-risk pregnancies to district or state hospitals. The ANM is assisted by a male health worker whose duties include motivating men to participate in the family welfare programme and also educating them about reproductive tract and sexually transmitted infections. The ANM and LHV also assist the medical officer at the PHC where health services, including antenatal and postnatal care, are provided (Government of India, 1998).

The National Population Policy, adopted by the Government of India in 2000, reiterates the government's commitment to the Safe Motherhood Programme within the wider context of reproductive health (Government of India, 2000). Among the national socio-demographic goals specified by the 2000 policy, several goals pertain to safe motherhood, such as 80 per cent of all deliveries should take place in institutions by 2010, and 100 per cent of deliveries should be attended by trained personnel. In Haryana, the percentage of institutional deliveries is only 18 per cent which includes public or private health facility and NGO/trust. Conversely, 82 per cent deliveries are either at women's own home or parent's home. Furthermore, the proportion of home deliveries in rural area is as high as 85 per cent. Regarding the assistance during the delivery, the NFHS-2 reports that only 42 per cent deliveries are assisted by doctors, ANM/nurse/midwife/LHV or other health professional whereas 58 per cent deliveries are assisted by traditional birth attendants (*dais*). Out of deliveries which are attended by *dais*, 75 per cent of them occur in women's own homes and rest of them in their parent's house (IIPS, 2001). Care by *dais* creates particular interest because of the contrast between the apparent attraction of maternity services provided by private maternity homes and state health care system, and reluctance to use state health services. Kumar (1999) in his study observes that the poor availability of health services in villages of Haryana deters the access of use of health services. Although there does seem to be a trend towards increasing use of institutional services in urban areas, but in rural areas women still regularly rely on *dais*. Institutional services, on the other hand, are more consistently utilized for child care and treatment of diseases. In comparison, observers elsewhere have noted that obstetrical services tend to attract clients more quickly than other services, due to the observed benefits of improved care (cf. Foster, 1962; Landy, 1977). Traditional treatment methods were held to be most relevant for treatment of the reproductive system – for impotence, sterility, and disorders of menstruation (Maclean, 1976). Thus, the present paper focuses on the following objectives:

- Why despite the tremendous efforts by government the people are not accepting the concept of institutional deliveries and assistance by professional nurses/ANMs/doctors/LHV/ midwife etc.
- To understand the context of change in birth practices by demonstrating that *dais* is a therapeutic system comprising a shared set of values, beliefs and practices.

## The Setting

The village of Dhandhlan is selected as a primary research site. The village is well connected with roads and communication system. Thus, the regular transmission of information that reports concerning obstetrical care alternatives get circulate, and women would be aware of the options available to them and have some basis of evaluating the various alternatives. Dhadhlan village seemed appropriate due to its location at the intersection of several settlements, housing, state maternity facilities, PHC and sub-centre. Thus, the village seemed to serve as an illustrative site to investigate the alternatives available to a woman seeking maternity care and to examine the factors involved in her choice of a *dai*.

Dhandhlan village is located in the Beri tehsil of Jhajjar district. The village accounts for 485 households. The literacy rate in the village is 71 per cent. Numerous caste groups inhabit the village, e.g., Jat, Brhahmin, Bania, Kumhar, Khati, Lohar, Nair, Chamar, Dhanak, Valmiki, etc. Scheduled castes constitute the 17 per cent of the total population. The economy of village is almost agricultural and supplies milk to the neighbouring areas.

## Methodology

Two sets of respondents have been taken for the study. At the first place all the 10 *dais* of the village have been taken for the in-depth interview. The sociological and career attributes of *dais* are recorded. *Dai* as a healer and how she carries out her work in the comprehensive perspective has been recorded. On the other hand, out of total 202 women in the reproductive age group in the village, 20 per cent (nearly 50) have been selected for narrating their experiences with *dais*.

## I

## Sociological and Career Attributes of *Dais*

Although all women are expected to have a general competence with reproductive disorders, pregnancy and delivery, certain women specialize in treatment problems associated with such conditions. Via this route, women may acquire renown and respect which are usually the province of men. In order to understand the significance of *dai* as a female professional specialization, it is necessary to consider first the implications of being a healer in rural Haryana and then, specifically, the recruitment and skill acquiring work, function and remuneration.

### *Dai* as a Healer

The *dai* may be a medicine person, respected for her power, or she may merely be a person who assists at deliveries, who may claim knowledge of a few more medicines than the average woman but the range of her skills and few more medicines than the average woman but the range of her skills and knowledge does not afford her the recognition of being powerful. As a skill, *dai* also fits into the larger category of healing.

Cosminsky (1976) notes that many ethnographic reports do not differentiate a specialized status of midwife from any birth attendant. In addition, the World Health Organization (WHO) also classifies together all birth attendants as 'traditional birth attendants' if they assist at deliveries but have no 'formal training'. Cosminsky, then, uses the term 'midwife' in reference to a position which has been socially differentiated as specialized status by the society. Such a person is usually regarded as a specialist and a professional in her own eyes and by her community. Henceforth, *dai* will be referred in order to avoid confusion with government birth attendant or ANM or midwives.

### Recruitment of *Dais* and Method of Skill Acquisition

*Dais* are interviewed regarding recruitment and method of skill acquisition in order to draw conclusions regarding the uniformity in recruitment and training of *dais* as a family speciality, and on variance among different *dais* in type of training and source of skill acquisition. In casual conversation, while 80 per cent village *dais* claimed that they have learnt the skill from their mother, remaining

20 per cent claimed that they have acquired it from their relatives. Similarly, they learnt the speciality of midwifery also from a grandmother or mother. These patterns are congruent with the patterns of child socialization customary to village practice. Thirty per cent of *dais* claimed to have learnt midwifery by means of apprenticeship. Most described the process of learning as 'observation', or carrying the box which contains medicine and cloth. One way of understanding recruitment of *dais* is to examine the prospective replacements of the *dais*. To this end, we asked them, 'Will your daughter be a *dai*?,' and if not, 'who are you teaching or planning to teach?' Only 20 per cent of *dais* who responded are planning to have daughter as an apprentice, and of the others who planned to take an apprentice, the choices included daughter-in-law.

When asked to specify the source of their healing knowledge, 30 per cent *dais* described an apprenticeship, whereas 70 per cent said that if a woman is competent and her mother or grandmother was a *dai*, she is suitable and likely successor to the position. The discussion of the apprenticeship suggested that young women are not appropriate apprentices. Thus, only one *dai* indicated that her three daughters, ranging in age from 15 to 20 were too young to discuss medicines. Correspondingly, most *dais* claimed to have menopausal or post-menopausal phase before assisting at an supervised delivery.

## *Dai's* Work and Comprehensive Care

The topic of a *dai*'s assistance at her own child's delivery was addressed because of the cultural norms idealizing modesty between a mother and daughter; propriety inhibits an adult woman from displaying her genitals in her mother's presence. Of 10 *dais* with whom this issue is discussed, one said the equivalent of 'charity begins at home,' 80 per cent said it is improper to treat one's own daughter, and one said she would give advice and suggest medicines but would not physically present in the room with daughter. Correspondingly, most women of reproductive age stated that it would be very rare to have one's own mother present at a delivery, in fact, it would be embarrassing and improper and a woman would 'eat shame' to have her mother see her nakedness.

The *dais* found to provide less comprehensive care than expected with regard to areas of specialization covered in her practice. They are expected to provide counselling with reproduction and treatment in areas of specialization theoretically associated with reproduction; thus questioning revolved around those areas of health care, with which a specialist in women's problems might possibly deal. In interviews *dais* are asked to describe the types of complaints they dealt with and they are questioned explicitly regarding the following subjects:

- menstrual problem;
- sterility;
- pregnancy and delivery;
- child care;
- nutrition.

Of all *dais* who responded to these questions, none claimed competence in all the suggested areas; only two specialized in one single area. The most frequent response is that the *dai*'s area of competence is pregnancy, childbirth and child care, particularly for children under three years of age. Two *dais*, in addition to treating pregnant women and children, also dealt with other types of complaints: one with illnesses caused by sorcery and the other with common ailments of adults such as cough and stomach disorders. An other *dai* dealt with problems associated with pregnancy and delivery, child care and menstrual complaints. One *dai* specialized in 'food counselling' for pregnant women with appetite problems during pregnancy and two *dais* handled pregnancy, child care and sterility problems. In sum, the core of the *dais* focuses on activities associated with pregnancy such as appetite problems or preventive medicine for possible complications during labour pains.

The *dai*'s role does not usually include diagnosis of pregnancy. Women state that some village women need to consult a more knowledgeable woman in order to determine whether it is pregnancy or sickness but other women do not. Diagnosis of pregnancy, then, generally fall within the realm of every woman's competence. Most *dais* can, however, tell if a woman is pregnant by observing the woman's breasts, skin colour, general appearance and, of course, stomach size. Pregnancy diagnosis is considered a very private matter and one woman, who had experienced some ambiguous signs which she supposed might indicate either illness or pregnancy, said that she did not consult the *dai* who delivered her last child, in order to diagnose her condition. Rather, she discussed her symptoms with an elderly woman in her husband's family in order to 'keep the secrets of the household in the household.' This statement might also indicate fear of sorcery against the unborn child by jealous outsiders.

### Remuneration

*Dais* are also interviewed regarding remuneration as part of a more general effort to elicit information on their social position and on midwifery as a speciality in comparison to other specialities. Remuneration, respect and other indicators of gratitude are considered to be indicative of the value attributed to the role of *dai* and hence to have implications for selection of birth assistance.

In contemporary times, *dais* may receive both money and produce or clothes in return of their services. However, remuneration is variable and very much dependent on the will, or charitability, of the clients and their families. Many *dais*, when asked about payment for services, remarked in disgust that some people forget what they owe you so quickly and they do not get. A salutation may be the only recompense a *dai* receives for preparing and administering medicines, and assisting at a delivery. Cosminsky (1976), in her review 'Cross-cultural Perspectives on Midwifery' stated that the midwife usually occupies a respected position but her status is not invariably a high one. The indigenous midwife in India, to list one instance, is held in low esteem due to beliefs regarding pollution. In contrasting the status of Bariba matrone, one finds examples of some customary modes of indicating respect such as praise-singing (for the greatly admired), and reference by the title 'medicine person', which suggest a high status for the matrone (Sargent, 1982: 73). Gifts system was intrinsic to the traditional feudal social organization. Some *dais* did state that although they are irregularly paid at the time of delivery assistance, and the mother of the daughter also gives presents to the *dai*.

## II
## Indigenous Practices of *Dais*

Questions are asked to *dais* regarding their indigenous practices. The intent of asking about indigenous practices is to determine the complications frequently encountered by them from amongst the complications which an obstetrician expects as a specialist in obstetrics to encounter and the range of treatments employed in response to complications.

## Cord Cutting

The practice of cutting the cord only after the placenta is delivered is traditionally observed throughout the Indian subcontinent. Almost all *dais* wait until the placenta is out before trying and cutting the cord. This is considered a strongly polluting practice, with one *dai* saying that it is a serious sin equating it to the killing of a 100 cows. Indigenous practitioners consider the infant-cord-placenta as a package. They have been together for nine months, cord and placenta functioning to nurture the foetus – why should they be severed too quickly? But *dais* handle these bodily parts and respect the function that they play in growing the infant.

*Dais* say that they use the placenta as a tool to revive an infant who is not breathing and that the placenta is easier to deliver if still attached. One *dai* reported:

> In hospital doctors have machines and medicines – here we do not have those means to deal with a new born who is not breathing – we need to be able to use what means we know.

## Placenta Cord

The cord is cut only after placenta delivery, and after the child cries. If cord is cut before placenta is out, it is harmful for the mother because the placenta may go up. The practice of not cutting the cord until the placenta is delivered is common in all the areas.

The act of cutting the cord usually comes across in anthropological studies as a highly polluting act and looked down upon as dirtying and degrading. In fact, a lot of young women from *dai* communities do not learn the *dai* work precisely because of these attitudes being held by society at large and their own aspiration for modern, higher status jobs. Again, this is where caste and gender biases intersect. The female body and the by-products of conception as well as the work of birth are denigrated. But *dais*, as mentioned above, handle these bodily parts and respect the function that they play in growing the foetus. One of the *dais* asserted:

She never cuts the cord, and that cutting the cord is a great sin, gives us a clue as to an impulse behind the distaste with which cutting the cord is viewed. Something alive (having *jeevan* or life) is being violated by being served. The moral right to perform that act is seen as the mother's prerogative. This assumes that the mother herself is aware, awake and an agent in the process of birth. Within her body the baby grew; she gave birth; and now it is she who has the role of finally separating this new life from her body.

## Energy *(Hawa-gola)*

After the baby is born, the vagina (*shareer*) is open. In our place a clean cloth is made into a thick pad, it is warmed and placed on the vagina, so that cold wind *(hawa)* does not come. After birth of the baby, woman has *gola* pains. Because when the baby is in the womb then *gola* is the protector of the baby. *Gola* is located beside the baby. After birth *gola* is left alone so it looks for the baby in the womb. And this gives pain to the new mother. Therefore, immediately we give warm *halwa* (sweet mixture made out of flour, sugar and ghee) to eat and this foments the *gola.* Warm pot is placed on the abdomen for fomentation. This eases her pain. *Hawa-gola* is considered as a threat to the woman's well-being postpartum. Our current understanding is that *hawa-gola*, often referred to together, is some kind of matter, force or energy which must come out of the body (through the vagina or birth canal), and by all means not go up into the upper part of the body. Thus, the concern about the placenta (*anwal)* going up in the body (medically speaking, a retained placenta). It seems that although the *dais* are literally referring to the placenta going up, they are signifying an energy of the body (i.e., that of growing the foetus) that must not be retained within the body. If the energy (*hawa-gola)* remains within the maternal body, then it is considered a cause for pathology.

Interestingly, one of the synonyms *dais* gave for *hawa-gola* is mother's love *(mamta).* Here is an active notion of the space the baby has occupied and the feelings of the mother for the child are connected to the biological process of pregnancy. The *gola* is 'the baby's home'. It 'searches for the baby' after birth. Interestingly, both sensation and perception are attributed to the uterus/woman. What in bio-medical language is termed 'involution' of the uterus, is considered a phenomenon experienced by the whole body/person. The pain of the contracting uterus is understood to be caused by this 'search' for the baby. The space which was previously occupied by the baby is now empty and must be dealt with or it will become a site for the pathology of *hawa-gola*.

### Bemata

*Bemata* is an old woman, has white hair and walk with the help of stick. She stays under the earth and make puppets and gives them to people. She gives to some people and does not give to others. When a baby smiles, it is believed that *Bemata* is making her smile. *Bemata* is a powerful and creative divine persona invoked at the time of childbirth, with some variation in names, throughout North India. She is the special patron of *dais* and parturient women, lives underground and creates beings out of earth – breathing life into them. She writes the destinies of the newborns, shortly after their birth. *Bemata* is immanent in all nature, grows and protects the baby in the womb, but also seems to be responsible for complications if she does not 'exist' the mother's body via postpartum bleeding. She is understood to leave the birth home at *chhatti* – and is thanked for growing and protecting the baby. But she is also sometimes blamed and held responsible for diseases of mother and child in the postpartum period. It is interesting that the presence of the same force which is seen as benign and fecund at one time (pregnancy and birth) becomes destructive and dangerous at another, post birth, if she/it is not in the process of diminishing or leaving. Thus, finally, the meaning of *Bemata* is entirely contextual and time-dependent. The concept encodes a process orientation towards birth and postpartum.

### Haemorrhage

Haemorrhage is bad blood which needs to expel. Air ball (*hawa-gola*) which is related to contracting uterus needs to be dealt postpartum. Putting baby to breastfeed immediately after birth works as a prophylactic against haemorrhage. This is not done because colostrum is considered bad for newborn.

## III

In order to determine the pattern of selection of birth attendants, 50 women are interviewed regarding person present at last delivery, neighbourhood of last birth attendant, etc.

## Person Present at Last Delivery

Of fifty cases reviewed, 48 per cent delivered their last child in the presence of mother-in-law or the 'old lady'. The *dai* is called for assistance in cutting the cord and/or supervising the delivery of the placenta. The remaining 52 per cent are assisted by village *dai* who not only helped in delivery of the child but also in cutting the cord and washing the baby.

## Meaning of Efficacy in Relation to Obstetrical Care Preferences

In the preceding pages, the argument was set forth that decisions regarding obstetrical assistance are influenced by cultural expectations, including generally shared concepts regarding the reproductive processes. Correspondingly, village women's expectations regarding appropriate sociological and career attributes of *dais* have implications for women's selection of a birth attendant. This section will focus on the village women's concept of birth as an event, the ideal behaviour for pregnant and delivering woman, and the implications of these expectations for the type of intervention which is likely to be considered necessary at birth based on the village women's definition of effective and appropriate obstetrical therapy.

In order to interpret the pattern of utilization of birth attendant among the village women, one needs to begin with the assumption that in choosing among alternative medical services, choices are ultimately based upon the perception and meaning of the services to the client (Riley and Sermsri, 1974: 52); the client also holds certain role expectations for the healer and acts according to the perceived meaning of the condition for which specialist intervention is sought. Thus, characteristics of the disorder, of the patient, of the healer, and of the services are all called into play as factors in decision-making with regard to obstetrical interventions.

Theoretically, all women are prepared to deal with a normal delivery. Pregnancy is not considered a disease, but rather a condition. One never hears referring to a woman being pregnant. When a woman is said to be sick during her pregnancy, the meaning is likely to be similar to what is referred to western medicine by the term 'coincidental illnesses of pregnancy' (Pritchard and MacDonald, 1976). Contrastingly, in western medicine, birth is considered a 'normal' physiological process but except under rare conditions, a delivery is a medical procedure. It is generally assumed that medical intervention is required at a delivery, whether or not complications occur. Frequently, pregnant women are classified by western physicians as low-risk or high-risk patients, but both require supervision, although different precautions would be taken for high-risk women depending on the problem involved (Pritchard and MacDonald, 1976).

A woman's knowledge of pregnancy is acquired not from healers who specialize in treating sickness but from more experienced women. A young married is informed by her grandmother and mother-in-law of cautions such as food taboos and prohibited behaviour which might harm the baby. A pregnant woman is likely to be told that she should work as hard as possible during her pregnancy so that at the time of delivery, her blood will not be thick and inhibit her from labour pain. If she feels contractions, she should ignore them, and keep working; her family should also pretend not to notice.

## Delivery at Institutional Clinic

To the village women, the delivery which most legitimately requires intervention is a complicated delivery. This category most often includes the women experiencing a problematic labour; the delivery is then termed 'not good', meaning not normal, e.g., a breech birth, child which slides on its stomach at birth, child born at eight months, etc. In such circumstances, woman is taken to institutional facilities. Here, the delivery is more public than a home delivery. However, usually, the woman delivers in a room with only the clinic personnel present; the relative or friend who accompanied her is not allowed in the room. In our study 90 per cent women asserted that the government midwife, especially when she is member of a different ethnic background, does not have the sense of belongingness and even not consider the individual person's ability to pay the fee.

In general, in comparing the roles of the village *dais* and the nurses/midwives/ANMs/, one overlaps in the provision of technical function. Both work towards the same outcome – delivery of the child. However, nurses/midwives/ANMs interpret the implications of birth more narrowly than do the *dais* and many of their clients. In the Dhadhlan village women describe *dais* as encompassing a complex of beliefs and practices not parallelled by the profession of ANMs/nurses/midwives/ doctors as practised in a clinic setting. The role of these institutional personnel is lacking in dimensions in comparison with the comprehensive technical, ritual and social functions of the *dais*. Informants criticized health services in institutional facilities as the staff behaves inappropriately to women in labour pain. From the perspective of clients, the alternative of institutional personnel for birth assistance cannot be selected because it could not be expected of them to solve the problem as defined by most village women. The village women say: '*Dais* are close to us, they dispense herbs, potions, massage and other familiar remedies on request and take time to provide conventional wisdom and personal services for people who speak the same language, both literally and figuratively, and often come from the same background.' They also reported that it is less expensive too. Increasingly, research on patient-practitioner relationships has demonstrated that decisions to select particular therapeutic options, and compliance with therapeutic regimes are influenced by the extent to which patients and practitioners share fundamental assumptions regarding clinical reality. This general conclusion has been thoroughly illustrated by Kleinman (1978); and for Africa, the review of health care systems by Good et al. (1979) has provided additional evidence that 'cultural empathy and value consonance between patient and healer' are of primary significance to therapeutic efficacy. Similarly, Dorothea Sich (1979) discusses obstetrics in rural Korea, where a rural health care project offered special emphasis on maternity care, including free midwife attendance. Nonetheless, project evaluation indicated that midwife attendance at birth had not risen substantially. Offered services in maternity care are not acceptable to the cultural conditions under which the recipients live. These conditions include the expectations that childbearing is a family responsibility, rather than that of the individual woman. The pregnant woman is not considered to be sick, and families disapprove of interference from outside. According to the village women, cosmopolitan medicine ignores or belittles the tenets of the indigenous obstetrical system, and the parturient women and their families hesitate to utilize the offered services, even when midwife/nurse/ANMs service is free of charge.

## Conclusion

Collecting indigenous knowledge of pregnancy and birth, the enthnomedical practices, concepts and beliefs associated with pregnancy, labour and delivery, the postpartum period, newborn care, obstetric emergencies, etc., is crucial to understand the decisions made by pregnant women, their families and the indigenous practitioners to whom they turn in times of pregnancy-related complications. What might seem irrational and a waste of valuable time to the biomedical provider and safe motherhood implementer, may be perceived as life-saving to the indigenous provider and the clients they serve. Indigenous birth practitioners (traditional birth attendants, *dais,* cord cutters, experienced family members and others) are locally available, culturally accessible, affordable and sustainable, and are appreciated by the women they serve. The indigenous system has the advantage of low cost, accessibility and sustainability. The methods are woman-friendly, low-tech and non-invasive. Clients experience mutual respect, shared cultural understanding and a continuum of care that is not possible in a medical set-up. Medical methods are perceived as invasive. Relatives, neighbours or friends are not permitted to participate in the birth. Familiar with birthing amid a circle of trusted women, women feel wretched when deprived of this. They report neglect and lack of care in government establishments. Private medical facilities charge high rates, speed up labour and undertake caesareans that may actually not be needed.

## References

Cosminsky, S. (1976), 'Cross-cultural Perspectives on Midwifery', in F.X. Grolling, S.J. Haley and H.B. Haley (eds), *Medical Anthropology*, The Hague: Mouton Publishers.

Foster, G.M. (1962), *Traditional Societies and Technological Change*, New York: Harper and Row Publishers.

Good, Charles et al. (1979), 'The Interference of Dual System of Health Care in Developing World Toward Health Policy Initiatives in Africa', *Social Science and Medicine*, 13D, pp. 141–54.

Government of India (1998), *Annual Report 1997–98*, New Delhi: Ministry of Health and Family Welfare.

——. (2000), *National Population Policy*, New Delhi: Ministry of Health and Family Welfare.

International Institute of Population Sciences (IIPS) (2001), *National Family Health Survey-2, 1998–99, Haryana*, Bombay.

Kleinman, Arthur (1978), Culture, Illness and Care: Clinical Lessons from Anthropologic and Cross-Cultural Research, *Annals of Internal Medicine*, 88(2): 251–258.

Kumar, Naresh (1999), 'The Provision of Infrastructure Services in Rohtak and Bhiwani Districts, Haryana, India, 1981–88: A Geographical Analysis', Durham: Unpublished PhD Thesis submitted to the University of Durham.

Landy, D. (1977), 'Role Adaptation: Traditional Curers under the Impact of Western Medicine', in D. Landy (ed.), *Culture, Disease and Healing: Studies in Medical Anthropology*, New York: Macmillan Publishing Co., Inc.

Maclean, Una (1976), 'Some Aspects of Sickness Behaviour among the Yoruba', in J.B. Louden (ed.), *Social Anthropology and Medicine*, Stanford: Stanford University Press.

Matrika (2000), *Crossing Boundaries and Listening Carefully: Empowering Women through Reclamation and Validation of Traditional Child-birth and Reproductive Health Knowledge*, Final Report.

Pritchard, J.A. and P.C. MacDonald (1976), *William's Obstetrics*, New York: Appleton-Century-Crofts.

Riley, J.N. and S. Sermsri (1974), 'The Variegated Thai Medical System as a Context for Birth Control Services', Working Paper No. 6, Mahidol University.

Sargent, Carolyn Fishel (1982), *The Cultural Context of Therapeutic Choice: Obstretical Care Decisions among the Bariba of Benin*, Dordrecht, Holland: D. Reidel Publishing Company.

Sich, Dorothea (1979), 'Traditional Concepts and Customs on Pregnancy, Birth and Post-Partum Period in Rural Korea', paper presented at First International Conference on Traditional Medicine, Canberra: Australian National University.

# 9 Medical Encounters

## The Experience of Illness and Treatment

The form and nature of the relationship between doctors and patients in medical consultations has been a popular theme for sociological study for many years (Bloom and Wilson, 1972). Since the early 1970s, however, concern has been expressed at the many shortcomings in that relationships, especially in consultation with women's reproductive health – that is, consultation occurring in gynaecological, obstetric and family planning settings where women interact with doctors about such matters as having or preventing babies, the menstrual cycle and female reproductive organs. Examining the functioning of the doctor-patient relationship in this context, sociologists have drawn attention to the medicalization of normal biological processes such as pregnancy and childbirth (Oakley, 1975), the control and dominance over decision-making exercised by the medical profession (Scully, 1980), and the poverty of communication between women patients and their predominantly male medical attendants (MacIntyre, 1981).

In this chapter we will discuss why medical sociological analyses of women patients' consultations changed from an acceptance of the medical model of events to a critical, consumerist view of interaction. In doing so we shall draw on observations of antenatal and postnatal clinics and wards, gynaecological clinics and wards, and family planning centres. We shall make use of interviews with the staff concerned, and with pregnant women contracepting women and infertile women in Rohtak city of Haryana.

## Historical and Political Contexts

Promotion of maternal and child health (MCH) has been one of the most important objectives of the family welfare programmes in Haryana. The Government of India also took steps to strengthen MCH. As part of the Minimum Needs Programme, initiated during the Fifth Five-Year Plan (1974–79), maternal health child health and nutrition services were integrated with family planning services. The primary aim at that time was to provide at least a minimum level of public health services to pregnant women, lactating mothers, and pre-school children (Kantikar, 1979).

In 1992–93, the Child Survival and Safe Motherhood Programme continued the process of integration by bringing together several key child survival interventions with safe motherhood and family planning activities (MoHFW, 1992). In 1996, safe motherhood and child health services were incorporated into the Reproductive and Child Health Programme. This new programme seeks to integrate maternal health, child health and fertility regulation interventions with reproductive health programmes for both women and men. With regard to maternal and reproductive health (MoHFW, 1997; 1998b), the important elements of the programme include:

- Provision of antenatal care, including at least three antenatal care visits, iron prophylaxis for pregnant and lactating women, two doses of tetanus toxoid, detection and treatment of anaemia in mothers, and management and referral of high-risk pregnancies.
- Encouragement of institutional deliveries or home deliveries assisted by trained health personnel.
- Provision of postnatal care, including at least three postnatal visits.
- Identification and management of reproductive tract and sexually transmitted infections (STIs).

The National Population Policy adopted by the Government of India in 2000 (MoHFW, 2000) reiterates the government's commitment to the safe motherhood programmes within the wider context of reproductive health. Among the national socio-demographic goals for 2010 specified by the policy, several goals pertain to safe motherhood, namely, 80 per cent of all deliveries should take place in institutions by 2010, 100 per cent deliveries should be attended by trained personnel, and the maternal mortality ratio (MMR) should be reduced to a level below 100 per 1,00,000 live births. Empowering women for improved health and nutrition is one of the 12 strategic themes identified in the policy to be pursued in stand-alone or inter-sectoral programmes. The low sex ratio in Haryana (i.e., 820 per 1,000 males) is mainly due to the sex-selective abortions despite the fact that Pre-Natal Diagnostic Technique (Regulation and Prevention of Misuse) Act was passed in 1994 (NFHS-2, Haryana). Medical Termination of Pregnancy (MTP) Act allows abortion in case of 'failure of contraceptive' but is silent about its use as a spacing method. Of the total MTPs recorded in India in 1990–91, about 42.2 per cent were done for failure of contraception (Chhabra and Nuna, 1994).

Concentrating women as mothers, their behaviour and social circumstances can lead to differential outcomes in reproductive behaviour like still births, infant and maternal deaths, prematurity, complications of pregnancy and so on. But, according to MacIntyre (1980), this perspective is limited in the sense that it reflects failure at the part of women's behaviour and exclude the organizational and other failures in the services themselves.

However, in the mid-seventies, sociologists began to question medical orthodoxy and with it the existence and operation of health services and the role of the medical profession within them. Some feminist groups and sociologists felt that doctors were making the natural, normal physiological processes of reproduction – conception, contraception, pregnancy and childbirth – into medical events to be actively managed and controlled by medical experts, who were alienating women in the process.

Two important and related themes can be identified in this theoretical critique of reproductive machine. First, a historical shift from female-dominated midwifery to male-dominated obstetrics was held to be the result of medical imperialism; that is, a tendency for the medical profession to expand its sphere of competence to include more and more new areas hitherto deemed outside its remit (Porter, 1990). Many examples of this tendency have been identified; mental health (Szasz, 1971), hyperactivity (Conrad, 1975), the care of old people (Illich, 1975). In the case of human reproduction it is argued that greedy, selfish and careless men expropriated from caring and careful midwives and lay women the power to help women reproduce naturally, joyfully and safely (Ehrenreich and English, 1973; Donnison, 1977; Oakley, 1976; Versluysen, 1981). Gynaecology and family planning were similarly seen as having been taken over by medical men with questionable motives (Scully, 1980; Roberts, 1981).

The second theme is related to the first and concerns the medicalization of reproduction. It has been argued that women and obstetricians have 'competing ideologies of reproduction': women seeing pregnancy as natural, normal, and a pleasurable life experience and doctors seeing it as a potentially pathological clinical event to be medically managed and controlled (Comaroff, 1977; Graham and Oakley, 1981; Nelson, 1983). This explains the medical profession's provision of antenatal care for what is essentially a normal state of health, doctor's preference for universal hospitalization at birth and active intervention in the form of induction and acceleration of labour, and for operative deliveries (Cartwright, 1979; Tew, 1986). Obstetricians' reliance upon medical technology and active intervention was seen as taking away women's control and their pleasure in reproduction and making them dependent on man-made machines and obstetric expertise. Birth was seen as having become unnatural, controlled and alienated (Fleury, 1967; Oakley, 1975; Cartwright, 1979). Katona's (1981) review of antenatal education led him to conclude that antenatal literature is geared to making women conform to this medical model of childbirth.

Similarly, it was argued that since the invention of the pill and the intra-uterine device (IUD) and the widespread decline in popularity of barrier methods which accompanied this, the provision of contraception was medicalized (Porter, 1986). Despite arguments that medical prescription was totally unnecessary, the most effective methods of contraception were under medical control. Doctors continued to resist attempts to make the pill available over the counter (Family Planning Association Conference, 1976) whilst denying women free choice of methods (Rakusen, 1981). Recently, it has been argued that the growth of infertility clinics and complex methods of infertility treatment have led to a medicalization of conception as well as contraception and childbirth (Arditti et al., 1984; Roberts, 1981).

Implicit in both these themes is the notion of a dominant medical profession which exercises control over the means of production – access to procedures, technology, information and so on – and thereby controls women's bodies and ultimately their lives. Much criticism of this medical dominance was to be found in the feminist health books which flourished in the mid to late 1970s (MacKeith, 1976; Phillips and Rakusen, 1978) which informed women how to deal successfully with the medical profession as well as to cope with the medical problems. In these works there was a great deal of criticism of the way in which doctors had hitherto dealt with women patients as having little understanding or sympathy for women with unwanted pregnancies, period problems, prolapse, menopausal problems, and so on (Daly, 1979; Ehrenreich and English, 1979).

Sociologists tended to concentrate on pregnancy and childbirth perhaps because of growing public and governmental concern with the functioning of the maternity services. Among women many criticisms of the maternity services were the impersonal: production-line atmosphere of antenatal clinics, their lack of continuity of care, their long waiting times and brief examinations, insufficient information, and no opportunity to raise problems or discuss progress (O'Brien and Smith, 1981; Graham and McKee, 1979; Oakley, 1979; Reid and McIlwaine, 1980). Intrapartum care was similarly criticized, with women being particularly dissatisfied with the lack of information provided to them, lack of choice and involvement in decision made on their behalf, and the unwanted and possibly unnecessary use of procedures such as shaving, administration of enemas, episiotomies, and pharmacological or mechanical intervention in labour and delivery (Cartwright, 1979; Oakley, 1980; Kirke, 1980; Boyd and Sellars, 1982).

In other words, research on women's experiences of reproductive health care suggested that the medicalization of reproduction was indeed experienced by women as alienating, that some use of technology and intervention was seen as unnecessary, that there were tremendous problems in communications between women patients and their doctors, and that medical dominance over information and decision-making in consultations was unsatisfactory for many women.

This change in attitude among patients and sociologists has been widely noted (Chalmers, 1978; MacIntyre, 1980; Hall et al., 1985), and various reasons have been put forward to explain it. Hall et al. (1985) have suggested that the many changes in technology relating to reproduction – ultrasonic scans, foetal heart monitors, epidural anaesthesia, and so on – which had occurred since the 1960s had been merely embraced but actively promoted by the medical profession. These changes occurred at a time when the ecology movement was promoting the 'natural'; the anti-medical establishment lobby (embodied by Illich, 1975) was fashionable; and the consumer movement was calling for more evaluation and control of services and a more caring attitude.

## Sources of Data

Direct observation is a particularly useful technique where detailed description of behaviour and social interaction is required rather than respondents' opinions of what they are doing or what is going on in a situation. There may be some differentiation between practitioners' accounts of their behaviour and their actual behaviour. Doctors, who were interviewed in the study of antenatal care, for instance, expressed concern over the poor quality of their patients' experiences at overcrowded and impersonal antenatal clinics, giving women very little opportunity for discussion. Equally, many doctors may believe that they have changed their attitudes and behaviour in the consulting room as a result of public criticisms much more than they actually have. This would not be apparent if reliance was placed solely upon interview material.

Providing that observers are accepted in the situation studied, the data collected can be very rich, consisting not only of description of events and social processes but also recording invaluable conversations with those observed. During periods of observation medical staff also made off-the-record comments about patients or their practice frequently.

The units of investigation were those patients who visited the antenatal clinics, family planning clinics, gynaecological wards/clinics and maternity homes. The medical doctors, paramedical staff, midwives, health visitors, nurses, receptionists and so on have also been observed and interviewed in a number of different settings.

## Analysis

We have sufficient data to examine the different aspects of reproductive health consultations in relation to gynaecolgy, antenatal check-ups, and family planning consultations whether they occurred in hospitals, maternity homes, or patients' homes. These will be discussed under medicalization, communication, and medical dominance.

## Medicalization of Reproduction

Medicalization in the reproductive process has increased tremendously over a period of time. New techniques have been introduced for the treatment of infertility. There has been rapid growth of infertility treatment clinics – clinics to identify the health of baby in the womb, clinics for the observation, etc. On the other side the government has decreased the outlays for health services in the public sector and has given path for investment to the private and corporate houses in medical service sector. It has also given way to the more medicalization of routine health affairs. In a small city of Rohtak itself there are more than 50 doctors who are practising as gynaecoligists, more than 20 maternity homes, two big hospitals and number of small establishments.

Apparently, in recognition of women's feelings about and preference for those delivering antenatal care there have been devolution of powers from obstetricians to midwives and doctors, and a movement away from specialist's hospital clinics to community health centres. This is because they found that doctors in private clinic provide service in a more friendly and personal manner. In the rural setting most of these affairs are managed by female health visitor or midwives, but respondents did not perceive any great benefit in the midwife's care and did not think she had done anything extra which the doctor could have done it. On the whole, this implies that whether it is a doctor of a specialized hospital, or of private nursing home, or midwives, the pregnancy is still seen not only in medical terms but is also managed medically and not as a natural, normal event.

There is an incident which we have recorded during our observation between doctor and the woman with her first pregnancy:

> Doctor: (after checking the position of foetus) You should take rest as the baby is not growing as fast as it should.

Patient: Than what to do?

Doctor: Really it is a serious matter, therefore, you should stay here till the baby is born.

Patient: It is very difficult for me to stay here till the baby is born.

Doctor: You see on the ultrasound the baby is not growing well and in other tests also there is deficiency.

Patient: If my husband wants to come and talk to you about inducing me, can I call him?

Doctor: I do not think anything your husband said would affect our decision one way or other way.

Patient: But he would like to talk to you.

Doctor: Yes, well he can talk to whosoever is on duty, but there is nothing he can say that will affect us. It is a medical question.

Patient: I understand it, but still he would like to talk to you.

Doctor: If we explain to everyone, and everyone's husband, we would spend all our time in explaining. I think you have got to assume if you come here for medical attention that we make all the decisions.

The doctor starts by giving a rudimentary account of why she wants to induce labour. This is offered in 'lay' language. It is apparent that her decision is made and she has no wish to discuss it. When the patient resists, she introduces 'technical' terms – ultrasound, etc. Graham and Oakley (1981) write: 'Technical language in explanations is reserved for cases where a doctor wants to encourage a patient to agree to a particular procedure (and perceives her as unwilling to do so)'. This is an example of manipulation, where the doctor employs speech acts for their perlocutionary effects.

Further, our study also finds the subjects who objected to induction all met with hostility. Women who explicitly or implicitly requested an induction met with a different response: 'In some cases the patient's request was granted, but even when it was not, the plea for induction was accepted as legitimate patient behaviour. They suggest that women who ask for an induction are subscribing to two important norms in obstetric practice: the idea that technological childbirth is good childbirth, and the notion that while the doctor's superior expertise may be challenged by refusing medical decisions, it is confirmed by polite requests for them; *begging for mercy,* etc., which doctors often describe.'

## Communication

Generally, the Family Planning Unit at Medical College Hospital, Rohtak has women doctors. We observed that they are often impatient with women's difficulties and doubts about their contraceptive methods. Junior women doctors are just as likely as men to make unkind or sexist comments about patient or lack understanding of their problems. The following conversation occurred between a female who has come to discuss her menstrual cycle problem:

> Female: Doctor, I have problem of irregular periods.
>
> Doctor: I too have the same problem, but still I come for work, so why did you take it seriously.

The doctor has no sympathy for the patient as she herself is facing the same problem. The other doctors of the unit also justified the doctor's reply as this is the correct attitude to pacify the patients.

Observing in gynaecology ward and clinic we noticed the doctors still tend to label certain patients for whom they cannot find a solution. Women with undiagnosed and pelvic pain tended to be labelled as 'fussy'. One doctor explained to us:

> Women come with their projected problems in their daily lives on to their pelvic organs and appeared at the clinic with unspecified.

Similarly, doctors at Family Planning Clinic tended to label women who had tried but could not find a satisfactory method of contraception as 'something uncomfortable' and to be visibly impatient with them. Although the doctors acknowledge that

> all methods have flaws and the choice for some women is very small, they think that the normal, reasonable woman ought to be able to find something to suit her.

Thus, the labelling of problematic patients is common by doctors as they believe that we also do not live in an ideal-type situation. Our observation shows that doctors still tend to disbelieve patients if their explanation or information does not fit with the doctor's own assessment of the situation. Following is the observation:

> Doctor asked patient when you did last intercourse without contraception. Patient said never. Doctor shouted at her. Doctor is not ready to accomplish the failure of contraception.

Doctors' view of procreation seemed to have changed little since MacIntyre (1976) described, 'Social construction of instincts – namely, the notion that married women instinctively want children and unmarried women do not. Thus, the young married women who claimed to have conceived the first time even having the protected intercourse is less likely to be believed by the doctors'.

In antenatal clinics, pregnant women are still treated as unreliable observers of their menstrual cycles, and therefore, doctors prescribe certain tests and scans for exact gestation of pregnancy rather than the woman's recollection of her last menstrual period. Doctors seemed unaware of the distress it could cause a woman suddenly to find her pregnancy put back a month because her dates did not agree with the scan and test. Similarly, contracepting women are also not treated as reliable witness to the side effects they experienced. Weight gain, depression, loss of libido are often put down to women's lives rather than the effects of the contraception pill.

On quite a number of occasions women raised questions which are simply ignored by doctors because, it seemed to us, the question is not defined as relevant by the doctor. The patient in the following situation is referred to the gynaecology ward with menstrual irregularity:

> Patient said that one of the menstrual problems is that after periods that everything is falling out. Doctor said, D and C will not do anything at this stage. Doctors discussed about the medicines she has been taking. Patient said that in these days I am feeling shaky and doing nothing. Doctor said she will give some tablets and explain how to take them. Since the patient is not literate, therefore, she asked doctor to write the tablet and instructions as the verbal instructions will be forgotten by her. Patient asked if shaking is due to the change of life. Doctor said that the menopause will not cause her to be shaky and then described the healthy condition of her cervix.

In another case women referred with menstrual problems mentioned intolerable side effects of some contraceptive method they have been using or the length of time they have been trying for a family without success. Some doctors ignored such 'irrelevancies' completely, whilst others acknowledge but did not explore them. Thus, behaviour is contrary to modern notions of good medical practice, as analyses of doctor-patient communication have long stressed the importance of hidden agenda, particularly in consultation of the sort (Zola, 1963; Balint, 1964). Thus, the data suggest that knowledge sharing is very much restricted among the doctors. At the same time, no doctors suggested the patient for some self-examination, so the medicalization process is reduced.

## Medical Dominance

Poor communication or restriction in knowledge sharing is still occurring within reproductive health care. The medical profession also controls access to the means of reproduction – contraception, conception, abortion, sterilization, pregnancy and childbirth. This medical dominance operates at two levels: First, doctors have the power directly to deny women access to procedures such as abortion, sterilization, treatment such as hormone replacement therapy and infertility drugs or methods of contraception and assisted contraception. Second, they are in a position to do so indirectly by limiting the range of options from which women may choose. This practice is particularly prevalent in family planning clinics where doctors not only with a stereotype of suitable patients, imposing their target-oriented methods of family planning in such a way as to deny women's choice.

The doctors often work with pre-notions of ideal-type patients. As a result, they offer certain women certain methods of contraception and withhold information for other methods. The following situation has been observed in the gynaecology ward:

> Doctor said the sterilization is best method as you do not to bother for fear of conception. Your husband will also not have any problem in intercourse.

From a medical point of view, second trimester abortions involve more risks of complications because of physiological reasons compared to the first trimester abortions. However, India ranks among countries with the largest number of second trimester abortions. Of the total MTPs recorded in 1990–91 for India, the share of second trimester MTPs was 15.69 per cent (cf. Chhabra and Nuna, 1994: 42). According to a community-based study in Maharashtra, about 29.1 per cent of the abortions were second trimester (Ganatra et al., 1997: 8).

Few providers also acknowledged malpractices that their fellow practitioners are engaged in, which caused women to face second trimester abortion. This included their lack of expertise and use of irrational drugs such as EP Forte, and involvement in providing abortion services by unqualified health personnel and general practitioners without a licence to provide medical termination of pregnancy.

One of the providers of the technique of ultra-sonography revealed its utility for individual's right as well as for the population control for the society. He commented:

> When there are techniques available for sex determination, why one should not do it? Otherwise what is the use of these (sonography) machines? ... The government should allow it openly.

Family planning consultants emphasized the good aspects of methods they approved and played down their shortcomings. This was particularly noticeable with respect to the sterilization method for females favoured by the majority of doctors. Women who asked about the risks or side problems are often told not to worry because for stopping the risks of contraception is the most important.

Another woman has come to the doctor for consultation of contraceptive method for short duration:

> Doctor said, you should go for pills. I would not advice you to use other method as they might bring infection and subsequently infertility. Infertility is a disaster particularly in the Indian families. It is directly related to the status of women in the family.

Thus, the woman who had her apprehensions about pills are dismissed by doctor. The woman had to rely on pills and forgo her own judgment. Such a situation reflects that family planning doctors are indirectly controlling women's access to methods of contraception and effectively limiting choice for the women.

Similarly, the access to abortion is also very limited, although the legal provision grants the permission for all the women to have the accessibility of abortion. But, in the real situation, doctors ask so many personal questions before providing such an access to women. The fear of non-medical enquiry by the doctor prompt many women to go for abortion. Many time doctors took the opportunity to lecture women for having repeat abortions or on sleeping around. This situation is observed as follows:

> The doctor asks the patient if she has guilty feeling after her termination. She said that she has but knew it is the best option to do so. The doctor pointed out the risk of termination and risk of infertility. Doctor advised her some methods of contraception for her future safety.

The significance of providers' perceptions and attitudes is evident when viewed against the fact that according to the MTP Act, it is the medical doctor who decides whether or not an abortion seeker fulfils the criteria spelled out in the Act. It is for the medical professionals to decide as to how liberally or restrictively to interpret the Act in a given socio-political context.

In this context, in one of the situations, the provider of the abortion service mentions:

> It is not their job to prevent unwanted pregnancies. We do not counsel for post-abortion contraception. Women's repeat abortions because of non-use of contraception for spacing had earned abortion providers their business. More frequent abortions increase our income.

## Conclusion

The foregoing discussion suggests that women's experiences in the reproductive health consultations have not changed in the medical profession. The medical profession does not define the childbirth and pregnancy process as natural and normal. On the contrary, demand for expansion of pre-pregnancy care and routine use of antenatal clinics suggests that medical domination of women's lives and lifestyles is increasing. Not only does medicalization of reproductive health continue virtually unabated, but also communication between patients and doctors often remains poor and the dominance of the profession over information and decision-making is unremitting. Consultation would need to change both their content and form much more in order to satisfy the critics of the medical profession.

## References

Arditti, R., R. Klein and S. Minden (eds) (1984), *Test-Tube Women: What Future for Motherhood?*, London: Pandora.

Balint, M. (1964), *The Doctor, his Patient and the Illness*, London: Pitman.

Bloom, S. and R. Wilson (1972), 'Patient-Practitioner Relationships', in H. Freeman, S. Levine and L. Reeder (eds), *Handbook of Medical Sociology*, Englewood Cliffs, NJ: Prentice-Hall.

Boyd, C. and L. Sellars (1982), *The British Way of Birth*, London: Pan Books.

Cartwright, A. (1979), *The Dignity of Labour? A Study of Childbearing and Induction*, London: Tavistock.

Chalmers, I. (1978), 'Implications of the Current Debate on Obstetric Practice', in S. Kotsinger and J. Davis (eds), *The Place of Birth*, Oxford: Oxford University Press.

Chhabra, R. and S.C. Nuna (1994), *Abortion in India: An Overview*, New Delhi: Veerendra Printers.

Comaroff, J. (1977), 'Conflicting Paradigms of Pregnancy: Managing Ambiguity in Antenatal Encounters', in A. Davis and G. Horobin (eds), *Medical Encounters: The Experience of Illness and Treatment*, London: Croom Helm.

Conrad, P. (1975), 'The Discovery of Hyperkinesis: Notes on the Medicalization of Deviant Behaviour', *Social Problems*, Vol. 23, pp. 12–21.

Daly, M. (1979), *Gyn/Ecology: The Metaethics of Radical Feminism*, London: Women's Press.

Donnison, J. (1977), *Midwives and Medical Men: A History of Interprofessional Rivalries and Women's Rights*, London: Heinemann Educational Books.

Ehrenreich, B. and D. English (1973), *Witches, Midwives and Nurses: A History of Women Healers*, London: Writers and Readers Publishing Cooperative.

——. (1979), *For Her Own Good: 150 Years of the Experts' Advice to Women*, London: Pluto.

Family Planning Association Conference (1976), 'The Pill on or off Prescription?', 23 March, London: Family Planning Association.

Fleury, P. (1967), *Maternity Care: Mothers' Experiences of Childbirth*, London: Allen and Unwin.

Ganatra, B.R.S.S. et al. (1997), 'Induced Abortion in a Rural Community in Western Maharashtra: Prevalence and Patterns', unpublished manuscript.

Graham, Hilary and Lorna McKee (1979), *The First Months of Motherhood*, London: Health Education Council.

Graham, H. and A. Oakley (1981), 'Competing Ideologies of Reproduction: Medical and Maternal Perspectives on Pregnancy', in H. Roberts (ed.), *Women Health and Reproduction*, London: Routledge and Kegan Paul.

Hall, H., S. MacIntyre and M. Porter (1985), *Antenatal Care Assessed*, Aberdeen: Aberdeen University Press.

Illich, Ivan (1975), *Medical Nemesis: An Exploration of Health*, London: Calder and Boyars.

International Institute of Population Sciences (IIPS) (2001), *National Family Health Survey, Haryana, 1998–99*, Mumbai.

Kanitkar, Tara (1979), 'Development of Maternal and Child Health Services in India', in K. Srinivasan, P.C. Saxena and Tara Knitkar (eds) *Child in India*, Bombay: Himalaya Publishing House.

Katona, C. (1981), 'Approaches to Antenatal Education', *Social Sciences and Medicine*, Vol. 152, pp. 25–33.

Kirke, P. (1980), 'Mothers' Views of Obstetric Care', *British Journal of Obstetrics and Gynaecology*, Vol. 87, pp. 1029–33.

MacIntyre, S. (1976), 'Who Wants Babies? The Social Construction of Instincts', in D. Barker and S. Allen (eds), *Sexual Divisions and Society*, London: Tavistock Publications.

——. (1980), 'Review Article: The Sociology of Reproduction', *Sociology of Health and Illness*, Vol. 2, pp. 215–22.

MacIntyre, A. (1981), *After Virtue: A Study in Moral Theory*, London: Duckworth.

MacKeith, N. (1976), *Women's Health Handbook: A Self Help Guide*, 16 Methley Terrace, Leeds.

Ministry of Health and Family Welfare (MoHFW) (1992), 'Plan and Implement MCH Services', *National Child Survival and Safe Motherhood Porogramme*, pp. 27–29.

——. (1997), *Maternal Health Programme*, New Delhi: Department of Family Welfare.

——. (1998b), *Maternal and Reproductive Health*, New Delhi: Department of Family Welfare.

——. (2000), *National Population Policy 2000*, New Delhi: Department of Family Welfare.

Nelson, M. (1983), 'Working Class Women, Middle Class Women and Models of Child Birth', *Social Problems*, Vol. 30, No. 3, pp. 284–97.

Oakley, A. (1975), 'The Trap of Medicalized Motherhood', *New Society*, Vol. 34, No. 689, pp. 639–41.

——. (1976), 'Wise Woman and Medicine Man: Changes in the Management of Child Birth', in J. Mitchell and A. Oakley (eds), *The Rights and Wrongs of Women*, Harmondsworth: Penguin.

——. (1979), *Becoming a Mother*, Oxford: Martin Robertson.

——. (1980), *Women Confined*, Oxford: Martin Robertson.

O'Brien, M. and C. Smith (1981), 'Women's Views and Experiences of Antenatal Care', *The Practitioner*, Vol. 225, pp. 123–26.

Phillips, A. and J. Rakusen (eds) (1978), *Our Bodies, Ourselves: A Health Book by and for Women*, Harmondsworth: Penguin.

Porter, M. (1986), *Free to Choose? A Study of Contraceptive Decision Making*, Report submitted to Family Planning Association, London.

——. (1990), 'Professional-client Relationships and Women's Reproductive Health Care', in S. Cunningham-Burley and N. McKegany (eds), *Readings in Medical Sociology*, (pp. 182–210), London: Routledge.

Rakusen, J. (1981), 'Depo Provera: The Extent of the Problem: A Case Study on the Politics of Birth Control', in H. Roberts (ed.), *Women, Health and Reproduction*, London: Routledge and Kegan Paul.

Reid, M. and G. MacIlwaine (1980), 'Consumer Opinion of a Hospital Antenatal Clinic', *Social Science and Medicine*, Vol. 14A, No. 363, p. 8.

Roberts, H. (1981), 'Male Hegemony in Family Planning', in H. Roberts (ed.), *Women, Health and Reproduction*, London: Routledge and Kegan Paul.

Scully, D. (1980), *Men Who Control Women's Health*, Boston, MA: Houghton Mifflin.

Szasz, T. (1971), *The Manufacture of Madness: A Comparative Study of the Inquisition and the Mental Health Movement*, London: Routledge and Kegan Paul.

Tew, M. (1986), 'Do Obstetric Infranatal Interventions Make Birth Safer?', *British Journal of Obstetrics and Gynaecology*, Vol. 93, pp. 659–74.

Versluysen, M. (1981), 'Midwives, Medical Men and Poor Women Labouring of Child: Living-in Hospitals in Eighteenth-century London', in H. Roberts (ed.), *Women, Health and Reproduction*, London: Routledge and Kegan Paul.

Zola, I. (1963), 'Problems of Communication, Diagnosis and Patient Care', *Journal of Medical Education*, Vol. 38, p. 829.

# 10 Women and Mental Health

## Disposition, Narratives and Treatment

Today mental disorders stand among the leading causes of disease and disability in the world. One in four people in the world is affected by mental or neurological disorder at some point in his/her life. World Health Report (2001), which was dedicated to the theme of mental health, shows that these disorders are estimated for about 12 per cent of global burden of disease and also represent four of the ten leading causes of disability worldwide. It is estimated that 6.7 per cent of population suffers from mental disorders, together these disorders account for 12 per cent of global burden of disease and an analysis of trends indicates that this will increase 15 per cent by 2020. One in four families is likely to have at least one member with a behavioural or mental disorder.

Demographic projections suggest that mental illness along with heart diseases, AIDS and cancer will account for the top four illnesses around the globe very soon (Davar, 1999). The National Institute of Mental Health and Neuro Sciences (NIMHANS) in Bangalore estimated that two crore Indians need help for serious mental disorders, while a further five crore suffer from mental illnesses not considered very serious. These figures do not include neurological age-related progressive disorders such as Alzheimer's and Parkinson's. It also estimated that at least 35 lakh Indians need hospitalization on account of mental illnesses. But, the country has only 40 institutions that are equipped to treat patients suffering from mental disorders. Moreover, many of them are medieval-era, asylum-style institutions with high boundary walls and artificial barriers where patients are kept in solitary confinement (*India Today*, 11 July 2011). India needs at least 12,000 psychiatrists, whereas in actual position, there are only 3,500 registered psychiatrists in the country, which means approximately one psychiatrist per 3,00,000 people.

## Gender and Mental Health

Sex and gender both are important determinants of health. Biological sex and socially constructed gender interact to produce differential risks and vulnerability to ill health. Health cannot be fragmented or reduced to a single causal factor and women's mental health is no exception. Good mental health is intrinsically important conferring a subjective sense of emotional well-being on the individual woman and extrinsically important, representing a significant resource to the broader society in which she lives and works.

According to Mental Health Act, 1987, a 'mental illness' is a term used for a person who is in need of treatment by reason of any mental disorder other than mental retardation. However, in view of the amendments made in the Act, mental illness came to be known as a disorder of mood, thought, perception, orientation or memory which causes significant distress to a person or impairs a person's behaviour, judgement and ability to recognize reality or impairs the person's ability to meet the demands of normal life, with the abuse of alcohol and drugs, but excludes mental retardation. To understand the gendered mental health discourse, it is important to understand the social dimensions of mental health according to the 1981 WHO report.

'Mental health is the capacity of the individual, the group and the environment to interact with one another in ways that promote subjective well-being, the optimal development and use of mental abilities (cognitive, affective and rational), achievement of individual and collective goals consistent with justice and the attainment and preservation of conditions of fundamental equality'. This definition has several advantages in relation to women's mental health because it:

- stresses the complex web of interrelationships that determine mental health and the factors that determine health operate on multiple levels;
- goes beyond the biological and the individual;
- acknowledges the crucial role of the social context; and
- highlights the importance of justice and equality in determining mental well-being.

The definition does not mention gender, but gender can and does impact on the production of mental health at every social level – the individual, the group and the environment – and is critically implicated in the differential delivery of justice and equality. Gender configures both the material and symbolic positions women occupy in the social hierarchy as well as the experiences which condition their lives.

Gender is conceptualized as a powerful structural determinant of mental health. It interacts with its structural determinants including age, family structure, education, occupation, income and social support and with a variety of behavioural determinants of mental health (WHO, 2000). Understood as a social construct, gender must be included as a determinant of health because of its explanatory power in relation to differences in health outcomes between men and women. 'These asymmetries are manifested not only in terms of differential susceptibility and exposure to risks, for example, vulnerability to sexual violence, but also fundamentally, in the power of men and women to manage their own lives, to cope with such risks, protect their lives and influence the direction of the health development process. The balance of power has generally favoured men and relegated women to a subordinate, disadvantaged position' (Pan American Health Organization, 1995).

A gendered, special determinants model offers the only viable framework for examining evidence on all relevant factors related to women's mental health. From this perspective, public policy, including economic policy, socio-cultural and environmental factors, community and social support, stressor and life events, personal behaviour and skills, and availability and access to health services may all be seen to exercise a role in determining women's mental health status.

## Context

The relationship between women and mental illness is very complex. There is a gender inequality in every aspect of life, whether it is education, occupation, or any other situation. Inequality is practiced at every level including family, community and also at working place. The gender inequality in health is also sharply evident (Nagla, 2003). Davar (1999) analysed that at least one in five papers during 1990 made passing references to women and their mental distress. Indian data on women's mental distress and illness is not available. The studies on mental illness in the community (both rural and urban) show higher prevalence among women across the country. However, a comparison between males and females in the occurrence of severe and common mental disorders (in rate per thousand at risk of adult population) shows a higher prevalence of severe mental illness among males (13.10 for males vs. 11.50 for females) as opposed to common mental illness where the reverse is true (68 for males vs. 103.50 for females) (Davar, 1999). Severe mental illness is classified such problematic behaviour as found in schizophrenia, depressive psychoses, mania, epilepsy, mental retardation and organic brain syndromes whereas common mental illness includes major depression, hysteria, obsessive compulsive disorder, anxiety, phobia and somatisation disorders. Women are more likely to seek help from, and disclose mental health problems to, their primary health care physicians while men are more likely to seek help from specialists of mental health care and the principal users of in-patient care (WHO, 2001). Women very often use non-professional options for healing including exorcists, mystics, shamans, faith healers, etc.

As women underutilize most of the metal health services in India including hospital services such studies are not representative and very likely flawed. Another major problem can be a survey, which generates data by only questioning the head of the family, presumably the patriarch. Issac and Kapur (1980) showed that of the 313 cases of common mental health disorders, only 14 per cent were reported by families. The decision about providing health care to the members of a family usually rests with the male head of family. Social hierarchy in Indian families would ensure that women's health needs are neglected. Gender stereotypes regarding proneness to emotional problems in women and alcohol problems in men appear to reinforce social stigma and constrain help seeking along stereotypical lines. They are a barrier to the accurate identification and treatment of psychological disorder. Women are reluctant to disclose their domestic violence-related problems to their family members and also to the psychiatrist for the treatment. It often goes undetected.

Although overall there is little difference between men and women in prevalence of mental health problems, there are major differences in the prevalence of specific disorders, especially the more common ones. Both depression and eating disorders exhibit a marked female excess, whereas substance abuse disorders are more prevalent in men. Men have higher rates of completed suicide but women have higher rates of attempted suicide. Okuma and Shimoyama (1972) reported that male patients related onset of illness to problems in job performance and increased work responsibility, whereas a high incidence of problems concerning reproductive functions was noted by female patients. Reddy and Chandrasekar (1998) and Ganguli (2000) indicated high prevalence rate of mental disorders in the community, i.e., 58.2 per thousand. Twenty per cent patients, who visit any curative services such as dispensaries, health centres, hospitals or clinics for any reason, have significant psychiatric disorders (Shah, 1982).

## Gender Discourse on Mental Illness

Davar (2000) in her study looks at available data on the mental health of women in India from the multiple angles of theory, research, clinical practices and policy. She looks at epidemiological data on the prevalence of distress in Indian women and raises philosophical and methodological questions regarding the adequacy of available diagnostic categories. She makes a conceptual distinction between distress and illness. A pure biology-based illness model undermines the social aetiology of mental distress which becomes significant in the case of women. A majority of women suffer from distress that cannot be explained in purely medical terms. Davar offers a critical examination of the phenomenon of male aggression and its psychological impact on women. Categorization of male aggression, its regulating power on women, its high potential to injure and the social sexuality that it enjoys constitute a clinical problem. The aetiology of mental illness is also looked at in terms of culturally specific distress behaviour such as possession (by a spirit) and training. A topological analysis of culturally specific distress behaviour is useful in countering dominant western universalistic paradigm that often pathologies culture-specific phenomena. However, Davar cautions, cultural relativism need to be equally mindful of the reality of indigenous oppression. To valorize tracing and possession as symbols of protest against social marginalization is to gloss over the whole question of gender politics that determines the distribution of power with society. Metaphors are disguised communications and they do not have the power of social change which more realistic options available to men do.

## Objectives of the Study

The primary objective of this study is to argue for a greater emphasis on gender issues in mental health. Following objectives have been taken into account:

- Socio-demographic profile of mentally-ill patients
- Factors in the predisposition of mental illness
- Treatment and care of mentally ill
- Gendered nature of the mental illness

In analysing the role played by gender in shaping the prevalence patterns, an attempt is also made to explore risk factors, health-seeking behaviour, and access to treatment and care.

## Methods of Study

The District Mental Health Programme (DMHP) was started in the Kurukshetra district of Haryana in 1999 under the supervision of psychiatric department of Post Graduate Medical College of Rohtak. After the successful start of DMHP in Kurukshetra, two more districts – Hissar and Gurgaon – were covered in 2008. This study was carried out in the out-patient department of psychiatry, district hospital, Gurgaon. This is a secondary care health institution. Gurgaon district is situated in National Capital Region (NCR) and is about 32 km away from New Delhi, the national capital. Gurgaon has 12 Primary Health Centres (PHCs) and 75 Sub-Centres at rural level. Training programmes for medical officers and paramedical staff is a regular feature at psychiatric department of Gurgaon hospital. It is a part of DMHP guidelines.

All new 194 female patients of psychiatric disorders who reported to the department formed the study population for the present study. Patients' data is generated from those patients who had been diagnosed and treated in the psychiatric unit of DMHP, Gurgaon. Intensive interview was carried out with the patients and also with their relatives. Some narrations given by the patients about their life sequences/episodes are also presented in the form of case histories. Data were collected between May–June 2010. Since we do not have tools to measure the chronicity of mental illness, neither are we specialized in doing so, therefore, we thoroughly interacted with them and ascertained certain information in the form of episodes or certain other levels of information, although doctors call them the precipitating factors in causing the mental illness.

## Social Structure and Mental Health

Social structure is a concept used by social scientist's, particularly in the field of sociology and social and cultural anthropology, to refer to relationships or bonds between groups of individuals. The structure of society refers to the way society is organized into different parts: institutions, social groups, statuses and roles. The notion of social structure implies, in other words, that human beings are not completely free and autonomous in choosing their activities, but rather they are constrained by the social world they live in and the social relations they form with one another (Crothers, 1996).

Social structure presents an idea that society is grouped into structures with different functions, meanings or purposes. Family, religion, law, economy and class are all social structures. Closely related is the notion of social stratification, which refers to the idea that society is categorized into different strata, according to social distinctions, such as a race, class and gender. Social treatment of persons within various social structures can be understood as being related to their placement within the various social strata. For example, some argue that men and women who have otherwise equal qualifications receive different treatment at the workplace because of their gender. Others note that individuals are sometimes viewed as having different essential qualities based on their race and ethnicity, regardless of their individual qualities. When examined, these social distinctions are often considered stereotypes based on prejudice. However, these social distinctions often go unexamined because they appear to be the result of social structures rather than prejudices.

There are noticeable social structural differences between men and women; these differences have some biological roots, and they are related to the distinct social functions and social relations which men and women perform. The male-dominated societies provide advantages to males and try to perpetuate the subordination of women. These kinds of issues reduce women's agency because in this sense women have little choice or power in making decisions, and whatever choices are available are constrained greatly by the institutions, values and practices of the societies in which they live. Thus, on the one hand, women are faced with the victimization and subordination, and on the other hand agency, autonomy and empowerment are restricted by the structure of society.

The mental distress of women according to age group shows higher prevalence in reproductive years. Most of the studies break off at the age of 50 years or so. Among the studies that include old age, some showed a decrease in distress among women. However, it is also seen that widowhood brings in heightened mental distress. A study by Sandhya (1994) examines the forced changes in life after widowhood.

Table 1 depicts that in the age group of 20–30 years, there are 35 (18.04%) cases of the mentally-ill patients, and in another age group of 31–40 years, there are 92 (47.42%) cases. Thus, the majority of the cases are in the age group of 20–40 years, which is the most active and productive years in life. However, in the age group of 41 years and above, there are 67 (34.52%) cases.

Table 1 also shows the prevalence of mental distress and several other socio-economic variables. It is seen that the symptom rate is linked more with being married than being single. Being widowed, separated or divorced is also linked with a higher symptom rate. All the studies show greater distress in married women as compared to married men and greater stress in single women as compared to single men. Several studies have been cited

**Table 1** ***Socio-economic Profile of the Mentally-Ill Female Respondents***

| *Age Groups* | *20–30 yrs*<br>*35 (18.04)* | *31–40 yrs*<br>*92 (47.42)* | *41–50 yrs*<br>*53(27.31)* | *51–60 yrs*<br>*14 (7.21)* | *Total*<br>*194 (100)* |
|---|---|---|---|---|---|
| Marital status | Married<br>128 (65.97) | Unmarried<br>61 (31.44) | Widowed<br>5 (2.55) | — | 194 (100) |
| Education | Illiterate<br>64 (32.98) | Primary-12th Class<br>107 (55.15) | Graduation-Post-graduation<br>22 (11.34) | Professional<br>1 (0.51) | 194 (100) |
| Family | Nuclear<br>149 (76.80) | Joint<br>45 (23.19) | — | — | 194 (100) |
| Nativity | Rural<br>85 (43.81) | Urban<br>109 (56.18) | — | — | 194 (100) |
| Monthly income | Below ₹ 5,000<br>96 (49.48) | Rs 5,001–10,000<br>65 (33.50) | Rs 10,001– 20,000<br>17 (8.76) | More than ₹ 20,000<br>16 (8.24) | 194 (100) |
| Occupation | Housewife<br>124 (63.91) | Labourer/Class IV<br>60 (30.92) | Professionals (teachers, etc.)<br>4 (2.06) | Shopkeeping/Small Business<br>6 (3.09) | 194 (100) |

showing that marriage is a stressful occupation for women. Our study also shows that there are as many as 128 (65.97%) patients, who are married as compared to 61 (31.44%) who are unmarried. There are only 5 (2.55%) women who are widow.

Table 1 further depicts that there are 64 (32.98%) patients who are illiterate; 107 (55.15%) have education between the level of primary to senior secondary level; only 22 (11.34%) patients are either graduate or post-graduate whereas only one patient is having professional qualification.

Correlating mental illness with the structure of the family, it was noted by many of the studies that mental distress was much greater in nuclear families than joint families. Chakraborty (1990) found that joint families are perceived as fostering greater emotional bonding between members, as having more care givers to take care of the vulnerable and the weak, especially women and the elderly, and as being based upon mutuality and cooperation amongst its members. These studies led to an unabated hysteria among professionals after the 1970s that the greater fragmentation of Indian society into nuclear families will increase conflicts, stress and strains, particularly among the womenfolk. Sethi and Manchanda (1978) explain the greater stress among the female members in completely joint families as the result of the conflict emanating from the desire to loosen the traditional family ties. Chakraborty (1990) argues against romanticizing the joint family as these families engage in a process of positive selection thus excluding economically dependent or other vulnerable people. Since nuclear family is the trend of the urban society and Gurgaon is also regarded as high-tech city, therefore, 146 (76.80%) of our respondents are living in nuclear families and only 23.19 per cent are part of joint family system.

As in the case of family structure, the urban background is also reflected in the data gathered from the hospital. Little more than 50 per cent of mentally-ill women are from the urban background, and less than 45 per cent are from the rural background. Most of our mentally-ill patients are not working or in some cases even if they are working, they are engaged either as labourer or in lower class occupations. The income of almost 50 per cent respondents is below ₹ 5,000 per month. It may also be due to the fact that because of their poor economic background, they are in the government hospital for the treatment.

The illiterate, poor refugees, unemployed and women in low-paying work or sex workers, household maids and beggars are most vulnerable to mental distress. Studies in India have shown that even though fewer women get admitted to mental hospitals for care, the once they admitted they stay for a longer period of time. The reasons for this longer stay range from economic to the attitudes of hospital personnel towards them. Lobbying for easy discharge may be seen as aggressive and assertive behaviour, which is an indication that the woman has not recovered fully. An ideal woman patient is expected to be compliant, patient, passive, dependent and submissive. The data on occupations structure presented in Table 1 shows that majority of patients, i.e., 124 (63.91%) are housewives, another 60 (30.92%) are working as labourers or engaged in low-paid occupations. The data clearly depicts that only four women are professionals and working as school teachers or clerks and another six are doing very small business like shopkeeping, etc.

## Interests, Hobbies and Habits of Women

It is well known that if you are engaged in the activities which interest you, then, there are less chances of putting you in worries. Our study also found that a sizeable number of women do not have any specific interest or hobby. It may be because they are poor, depend on husbands and cannot afford to pursue their hobbies.

**Table 2** ***Interests and Means of Recreation of the Mentally-Ill Patients Before Hospitalization***

| *Interests/Means of Recreation* | *Number* | *Percentage* |
|---|---|---|
| Reading/writing | 2 | 1.03 |
| Television | 131 | 67.52 |
| Folk art | 11 | 5.67 |
| Listening of music | 35 | 18.04 |
| No special interest | 15 | 7.73 |
| Total | 194 | 100.00 |

Special interests, pursuits of leisure hours and certain habits help us understand the patient's pre-psychiatric personality in right perspective. Hence, an analysis was attempted. Table 2 brings out that the female patients are more accounted for television, i.e., 131 (67.52%) and lack other interests, thus, one gathers an impression that a considerable number of mentally-ill patients lacked adequate recreational interests and facilities.

## Factors in the Predisposition of Mental Illness

Mental illness arises from a complex interaction of genetic, biological, social, personality and environmental factors. Mental illness affects people of all ages, educational levels, and different cultures. Age, sex, substance abuse, chronic diseases and family and workplace situations and life event stresses are the major risk factors. In the present study we also analyse the risk factors that contribute to the mental illness among women. The 2003 WHO Report on Mental Health states that 'mental disorders occur in persons of all genders, ages and backgrounds. No group is immune to mental disorders, but the risk is higher among the poor, homeless, the unemployed, persons with low education ...' The link is, however, complex and is influenced by numerous factors. The socio-economic factors are associated with the risk for mental disorders. These socio-economic factors include poverty, deprivation, illiteracy and low household income. Being female is reported to be a risk factor for common mental disorders. Studies from India have shown that poverty and deprivation are independently associated with the risk for common mental disorder in women and add to the sources of stress associated with womanhood (Patel et al., 2006). Among women in poverty, there is support for a significant association between economic hardship and reports of psychological distress due to such issues as being the sole childbearing adult in a household, multiple roles, unequal power relations with men and a sense of powerlessness (Patel et al., 1999). Psychological factors such as low age at marriage, patriarchal structure of society, dominance of husband and domestic violence have strong association with common mental disorders. There is another important risk factor, i.e., the widowed or divorced. It is because it represents their social isolation and stigma. It also restricts their life in certain areas which in turn also adds to the mental illness. An analysis of the elements found active in the predisposition of depression indicates that several socio-psychological factors are common in many cases. Stresses and strains owing to psycho-social factors are observed to be responsible for mental illness. The significance of somatogenic and hereditary factors can neither be underestimated nor overstated. It is common that women have higher rates of anxiety and mood disorders, while men have higher rates of substance and impulse-control disorders than women. Gender disadvantage and exposure to intimate-partner violence are key risk factors for common mental disorders in women (Patel et al., 2006). Surveys have also shown an association between reproductive and sexual complaints (such as the complaint of vaginal discharge) and common mental disorders (Prasad et al., 2003; Patel et al., 2006). Younger age pregnancy, repeated pregnancy, son preference, multiple abortions, foeticide are all associated with common mental disorders. Besides these gynaecological problems like vaginal discharge, irregular menstrual periods and infertility are also associated with an increased risk.

**Table 3** ***Factors in Predisposition of Mental Illness***

| *Predisposition Factors* | *No. of Cases* | *Percentage* |
|---|---|---|
| Heredity | 17 | 8.76 |
| Toxins | 41 | 21.13 |
| Childbirth | 3 | 1.54 |
| Domestic worries | 109 | 56.18 |
| Sex and marital problems | 78 | 40.20 |
| Economic factors | 97 | 50.00 |
| Serious childhood problems | 21 | 10.82 |
| Bereavement of loved ones | 3 | 1.54 |
| Broken family | 17 | 8.76 |
| Total number of responses | 386* | 198.96 |
| Total number of mentally-ill patients | 194 | 100.00 |

* Answers in the multiple form.

Here, we will discuss the brief account of the social and cultural factors that work in the predisposition of depression. The theoretical viewpoints in regard to the causes of mental illness has been changing with the advancement of psychiatry. From the primitive man to the modern psychiatrist, mental illness has been attributed to a host of factors and to date, despite the highest scientific innovations and achievements, there is no finality of views regarding the causation of mental illness. In other words, each approach is researcher's orientation-oriented. A medical man tends to focus on the organic aspect of the illness whereas a psycho-analyst highlights the dynamics of some developmental phases. Sociologists will look into socio-cultural aspects of mental illness.

There are only 8.76 per cent cases where heredity has been observed in the predisposition of mental illness whereas, toxins in 21.13 per cent and childbirth in 1.54 per cent cases have been observed. Psycho-social factors, marital disharmony and maladjustment relating to the healthy development of the sex seem to be the greatest source of mental stress and strains. We find that 78 (40.20%) patients suffered from such problems. Besides, 97 (50%) faced economic problems, 21 (10.82%) had serious childhood problems, bereavement of loved ones was found in 3 (1.54%) cases, and problems of broken family in 17 (8.76%) cases led to mental illness (see Table 3).

## Clinical Manifestation among Mentally-ills

Table 4 clearly depicts that maximum number of mentally-ill patients have complaints of sad mood, poor appetite and loss of interest in usual activities. A sizeable number of mentally-ill women also thought of suicide or they wish to die.

**Table 4** ***Distribution of Clinical Manifestation among Mentally-ill Patients***

| *Clinical Manifestation* | *No. of Mentally-ill Patients** | *Percentage* |
|---|---|---|
| Mood | | |
| (a) Sad | 170 | 87.62 |
| (b) Irritable | 6 | 3.09 |
| (c) Fearful | 49 | 25.25 |
| Appetite | | |
| (a) Poor | 163 | 84.02 |
| (b) Loss of weight | 19 | 9.79 |
| Insomnia | 139 | 71.64 |
| Hypersomnia | 9 | 4.63 |

*Cont'd...*

...*Cont'd*

| | | |
|---|---|---|
| Loss of energy | 89 | 45.87 |
| Agitation | 23 | 11.85 |
| Loss of interest in usual activities | 192 | 98.96 |
| Guilt feeling | 93 | 47.93 |
| Complaints of or actually diminished ability to think or concentrate | 71 | 36.59 |
| Recurrent thought of death or suicide or death wish | 89 | 45.87 |

* Multiple responses.

## Treatment and Care of the Mentally-ill Patients

Each human ailment, physical or mental, calls for therapeutic attention. Some disorders are serious enough to warrant immediate therapy while others may not be so. However, the availability and type of curative treatment depend on many socio-economic factors and circumstances. In this context, we have asked the patients to mention about their pre-hospital treatment. It is pertinent to mention that all the mentally-ill patients have received some or other form of treatment from different indigenous or superstitious or magical men (sadhus, fakirs, etc.) except three.

**Table 5** ***Indigenous Practitioners who Treated Mentally-ill Patients Before Hospitalization***

| *Type of Practitioner* | *No. of Cases* | *Percentage* |
|---|---|---|
| Sadhus/Fakirs | 49 | 25.25 |
| Siyane | 53 | 27.31 |
| Hakims/Vaidyas | 73 | 37.62 |
| Elderly people of community | 3 | 1.54 |
| Cases who received treatment from indigenous faith healers only | 113 | 58.24 |
| Those who did not received any treatment at all before coming to hospital | 3 | 1.54 |
| Total | 294 | 100.00 |

A perusal of the earliest development of psychiatry unfolds that dogma and superstitious rites have had an intimate concern with the mentally sick since the dawn of history. In the primitive era, animism guided the treatment that the people with odd behaviour received through incantation, penance, religious ceremonies, suffering, torture, sacrifice, burning and flogging under the supervision of priests, etc. (Mohan, 1966). To date mental illness continues to be considered a manifestation of certain evil influences that possess the victim. Primitive beliefs and practices are widespread in communities, particularly those who are not illiterate or may be less educated. We found couple of healers who deal with the mentally sick people are: *sadhus* and *fakirs, siyane, vaidyas* and *hakims.* At times, we also found elderly persons, generally in village communities, dealing with the mentally sick. We found that 113 (58.24%) mental-ill patients have received treatment from the indigenous practitioners and only 3 (1.54%) did not receive any such treatment before coming to the hospital (see Table 5).

Types and methods of treatment received by the mental-ill patients before hospitalization phase are varied (Table 6). These include visits to and worshipping of a host of gods and deities as well as a number of practices typically characterized by crude and inhuman methods. In all, in 191 (98.45%) cases, patients received such treatment. In almost all the cases, except three, patients resorted to more than one type of treatment. The break-ups are worshipping of either deity 153 (80.10%), *tabeez* and *tona* 124 (64.92%), worship of some tree 63 (32.98%), *jhara* 78 (40.83%), *dhooni* 52 (27.22%), *hawan* 39 (20.41%) and herbal treatment of *hakims* and *vaidyas* 21 (10. 99%).

**Table 6** ***Type of Indigenous Treatment Received by the Mentally-ill Patients before Hospitalization***

| *Type of Indigenous Treatment* | *No of Cases* | *Percentage* |
|---|---|---|
| Worshipping of deities | 153 | 80.10 |
| Tabeez and tona | 124 | 64.92 |
| Worship of some tree | 63 | 32.98 |
| Jhara | 78 | 40.83 |
| Dhooni | 52 | 27.22 |
| Hawan | 39 | 20.41 |
| Herbal treatment of Hakims and Vaidyas | 21 | 10.99 |
| Total | 530* | 277.48 |
| Total cases | 191 | 100 |

*Answers are in multiple response form.

## Mental Health Policy

The National Mental Health Policy outlines the prioritized agenda for extending within a pragmatic time-frame basic mental health care facilities to all sections of the population across the country by the year 2020. The tactical vehicle for implementing the said policy will be the refocused National Mental Health Programme, initially formulated in 1982, with five key thrust areas:

(a) The District Mental Health Programme (DMHP), redesigned around a nodal institution which in most instances will be the Zonal Medical College.

(b) Strengthening the medical colleges with a view to develop psychiatric manpower (HRD), improve psychiatric treatment facilities at the secondary level and to promote the development of general hospital psychiatry in order to reduce and eventually to eliminate to a large extent the need for big mental hospitals with a huge proportion of long-stay patients.

(c) Streamlining and modernization of mental hospitals to transform them from the present mainly custodial mode to tertiary care centres of excellence with a dynamic social orientation for providing leadership to research and development (R&D) in the field of community mental health.

(d) Strengthening of central and state mental health authorities in order that they may effectively fulfil their role of monitoring ongoing mental health programmes, determining priorities at the ventral/ state level and promoting inter-sectoral collaboration and linkages with other national programmes.

(e) Research and training aimed at building up an extensive database of epidemiological information relating to mental disorders and their course/outcome, therapeutic needs of the community, development of better and more cost-effective intervention models, promotion of inter-sectoral research and providing the necessary inputs/ conceptual framework for health and policy planning. Focused IEC activities, formulated with the active collaboration of professional agencies such as the National Institute of Mass Communication and directed towards enhancing public awareness and eradicating the stigma/discrimination related to mental illness, will form an important component of this policy objective.

Recently, mental illness has been added in non-communicable diseases in the global platform in World Health Organization (WHO) conference held in April 2011. It pleaded its case that like all other non-communicable diseases, mental disorders also require long-term treatment and affect the quality of life. Skultans (1991) finds in her study of a traditional healing temple in western Maharashtra that women's mental afflictions are marginalized and stigmatized in comparison to men. Possession-trance, the activity whereby healing is primarily sought reifies '... the stereotypes of male fortitude and health and female weakness and ill health' ...

Then, the question arises, why do women stay away from psychiatry? It may be because of its social labelling and a social control function that is often claimed (Scheff, 1999; Foucault, 2001). Feminist scholars refute that mental illness treatment does not lie in women's minds and bodies (Dennerstein et al., 1993; Davar, 1999; Addlakha, 2001). Anthropological perspective views mental illness in its surrounding of local culture (Levy, 1992). However, Addlakha (2001) faces a dilemma when in Indian hospitals women are admitted with the issue of domestic violence. The psychiatrists contemplate their admission as a protection measure. In another situation, Nunley (1998) finds that families exercise a great control over defining the illness and its treatment course. Thus, it is not the system of spiritual healing or bio-medical treatment; rather both are gendered. For women in search of healing, both treatment facilities seem to echo and reproduce the larger patriarchal structures within microcosmic therapeutic practices (Skultans, 1991; Davar, 1999). To qualify our data more strongly for the interpretation of mental illness among women, we chose to strengthen them qualitatively with the help of some case histories of the mentally-ill women narrated to us during the process of our interview with them.

## Case Histories

In India, research has demonstrated the vulnerable status of women's perceptions of their rights. The study by Sharma et al. (1998) that more than 55 per cent women did not have power to refuse sexual activity. Another study by Khan et al. (2000) found that social, religious and cultural constraints serve to perpetuate the gender inequality and provide a type of justification for sexual abuse of women. Women are socialized to believe that they are inferior to men, and expected to serve and obey their husbands, and to satisfy their sexual needs (Chandra et al., 2003). Mentally-ill women are clearly among the least powerful members of society and are highly vulnerable to sexual victimization. Mental illness is also viewed as stigmatized disease particularly in India.

Some events occurred before the onset of mental illness when the women were living in the family. The description of case histories will enrich the qualitative findings in analysing the mental illness by putting the social context of depression, dependency and hopelessness in framework. The contributing or risk factors, which we have already discussed in terms of family breakdown, domestic violence, poverty and social pressures, result into the symptomatic behaviour of mental illness. Some of the narratives presented below revealed by the women in terms of the nature and severity of their experiences have resulted in the mental illness.

Muni was 14 years old, living with her married sister in her house. She was working as a maid servant in the nearby houses. Sister's husband was crazy about women. Her sister was also aware of her husband's character of eyeing towards other women, but she was helpless. Her sister never leaves Muni alone in the presence of her husband as she knows his habit. However, one day, her sister has to go to hospital as her younger son became ill. Muni was also out for work. When she returned from work, she did not find her sister there. Her husband got an opportunity and forcefully raped Muni. The woman is now suffering from psychosis.

### *Another woman reported on economic hardship*

Manju, a woman in her 30s, lost her husband in collapsing of wall at the construction site where he was working. He was a good worker and earning a substantial amount of money for meeting out their daily needs. Manju had three children. The sudden death of her husband has resulted in her shattered life and total despair. It was very difficult for her to cope with this tragedy and take responsibility of three children. In the family also she was unable to find a helping hand in this critical time. She many times thought of attempting suicide also. She is now suffering from depression.

*Another woman is victim of emotional deprivation*

Ranu, aged 23 years, lost her son in an accident. On the day of accident, Ranu sent him to bring milk. Since it was not very close to her house, therefore, she asked him to go on bicycle and bring milk but, unfortunately, he never returned. Now, she feels that she is responsible for his death as she sent him for fetching the milk. The accident disaster converged with the own guilt to culminate the fear of uselessness of life. She has an emotional deprivation because of his son's untimely death.

*Another incident of mental illness because of strong social pressure for son's birth*

Another woman, Sarita, age 22, reported that she has a strained relationship with her-in-laws and husband because of the strong desire for the male baby. She has three daughters, and when she became pregnant fourth time, her in-laws and husband insisted her for sonography to know the sex of foetus. When they came to know that it is again a female foetus, they forced her to get it aborted. They forcibly took her to doctor, and the doctor refused to do abortion. The abortion was risky as her health was not allowing her to go for abortion. Her husband's and mother-in-law's behaviour has suddenly changed. They started accusing and abusing her. Many times her husband hit her. One day he hit her so strongly that baby did not move for an hour and she thought it had died. After that she is scared of his hitting and abuses. This woman is now a victim of depression.

The case histories narrated above clearly reveal that the relationship of sexually coercive activity, poverty, emotional deprivation, and social pressure for giving birth to son has resulted into different symptomatic features of mental illness. As is evident by their narrations they suffered from different types of mental illnesses because of lack of judgment, disinhibition, and lack of self-awareness.

## Hospitalization and Treatment of Mentally-ill Patients

Out of the total respondents, there are 144 (74.22%) mentally-ill patients who are either dependent on husbands, parents, children, siblings or other members in the family. It is interesting to note that half of such patients, i.e., 72 (50%), are exclusively dependent on their husbands (see Table 7).

**Table 7** ***Dependency of Patients after Onset of Mental Illness***

| *Dependent on* | | | | | |
|---|---|---|---|---|---|
| *Husband* | *Parents* | *Children* | *Siblings* | *Others* | *Total* |
| 72 | 27 | 33 | 8 | 4 | 144 |
| (50.0) | (18.75) | (22.91) | (5.55) | (2.77) | (100.00) |

## Access to Treatment and Care

Despite the enormous disease burden of mental health disorders, treatment for mental health in most parts of India is grossly inadequate. Mental health research policy address women's health issues within a gender perspective. There are only epidemiological studies on mentally ills in India in 1970s and 80s that made some passing references to mental distress among women (Davar, 2001). The respondents are ill informed and do not know anything about it. There is a vast gap in their knowledge about the mental health treatment and policy at various levels.

Against this background, this part of the paper deals with the access to treatment and care for mental disorders. How women respond to their mental health problems? In India, persons with depression tend to be treated with a range of symptomatic medicines, such as analgesics for aches and pains, tonics and vitamins injections for fatigue and tiredness, and sleeping pills for insomnia (Patel et al., 2000).

## Admission into Hospital

Women very often use non-professional options for healing including exorcists, mystics, shamans and the like. When we look at our data relating to the admission process in the hospital, presented in Table 8, we find that majority of patients, i.e., 79(54.86%), have come to hospital of their own which means they are not referred or advised by private physicians or state post-graduate medical college, or other health care professionals. Another quarter of patients are old patients. It means they are already seeking treatment during our interview process. However, 21 (10.82%)

mentally-ill patients came to hospital as suggested by community leaders and the same number of patients are referred by other doctors of hospital.

**Table 8** ***Admission into Hospital for Treatment***

| *Referrals* | *No. of Patients (%)* |
|---|---|
| Through IEC | 4 (2.06) |
| Old patients | 58 (24.74) |
| Private physicians | 10 (5.15) |
| PGIMS, Rohtak | 1 (0.51) |
| Community leaders | 21 (10.82) |
| Other doctors in hospital | 21(10.82) |
| Self | 79 (54.86) |
| Total | 194 (100.00) |

**Table 9** ***Substance Abuse Among Mentally-ill Patients***

| *Substance Abuse* | *No. of Patients* | *Percentage* |
|---|---|---|
| Yes | 8 | 4.12 |
| No | 186 | 95.87 |
| Total | 194 | 100.00 |

**Table 10** ***Past History of Mentally-ill Patients***

| *Family History* | *No. of Patients* | *Percentage* |
|---|---|---|
| Yes | 28 | 14.43 |
| No | 166 | 85.56 |
| Total | 194 | 100.00 |

Since, our study is confined to the mentally-ill women, therefore, the data also corroborate that 186 (95.87%) patients are not having substance abuse or drug abuse history as majority of women in India are not in the habit of drug or substance abuse (see Table 9).

The past history of the mentally-ill patients suggests that only 28 (14.43%) patients were having the past history of mental illness. The majority of patients, i.e., 166 (85.56%), did not have any such past history of mental illness (see Table 10).

**Table 11** ***Type of Mental Illness***

| *Type of Mental Illness/Diagnose* | *No. of Patients* | *Percentage* |
|---|---|---|
| Anxiety neurosis | 16 | 8.24 |
| Bipolar affective disorder | 3 | 1.54 |
| Behavioural problem | 7 | 3.60 |
| Depression | 85 | 43.81 |
| Epilepsy | 34 | 17.52 |
| Somatisation | 14 | 7.21 |
| Schizophrenia | 17 | 8.76 |
| Migraine | 7 | 3.60 |
| Mental retardation | 8 | 4.12 |
| Obsessive compulsive disorder | 2 | 1.03 |
| Total | 193 | 100.00 |

Regarding the type of mental illness which has been diagnosed by the doctors, the data suggests that majority of patients, i.e., 85 (43.81%) are the cases of depression in contrast to obsessive compulsive disorder which is found in only two respondents. Nearly 18 per cent patients are victims of epilepsy, 16 (8.24%) are sufferers of anxiety neurosis and another 17 (8.76%) are schizophrenic. Similarly, 7 (3.60%) patients are suffering from migraine, and only 8 (4.12%) are having organic disorder, i.e., of mental retardation (see Table 11). Although, there is not much differences in the severe mental disorders like schizophrenia, but routine disorders like depression, phobia and anxiety are more common among women across all socio-economic groups (Sonpar and Kapur, 1999). Independent studies on mental depression across the world show that women are twice as likely as men to suffer from clinical depression (Davar, 1999).

**Table 12** ***Duration of Illness***

| *Duration of Illness* | *No. of Patients* | *Percentage* |
|---|---|---|
| 0–1 month | 19 | 9.79 |
| 1–3 months | 17 | 8.76 |
| 3–6 months | 19 | 9.79 |
| 6–12 months | 11 | 5.67 |
| 1–3 years | 58 | 29.89 |
| 3–10 years | 43 | 22.16 |
| More than 10 years | 27 | 13.91 |
| Total | 194 | 100.00 |

Finally, when we look at the duration of illness at the time of interview, we found that almost 30 per cent of mentally-ill patients were suffering for one year to three years. The duration of illness on first contact was between 3 to 10 years in 43 (22.16%) of the total patients. There were 13.91 per cent of patients who were suffering from more than ten years (Table 12). It may be due to the fact that they were not treated well at family, community, or at the level of different indigenous healers or health professionals.

## Conclusion

Gender is to be understood as an explanatory power in relation to differences in health outcomes and here in mental health outcomes between men and women. Mental illness affects women at younger age, and those who are married, illiterate or less educated, living in nuclear families, have urban background and are dependent on their husbands. Women's mental health is also determined by accessibility to mental health care, social support system, life events and gender stereotypes, etc. Domestic violence is the most potent factor found in the disposition of mental illness. Economic hardship, which also includes dependency on husband (as many women are not working outside), makes the women more vulnerable for mental illness. Sex and marital problems, childhood problems are also correlated with the mental illness. The mentally-ill women's behaviour is reflected in terms of their sad mood, poor appetite, and loss of interest in usual activities. A sizeable number of mentally-ill women also thought of committing suicide. Mental illness continued to be considered a manifestation of certain evil influences that possess the victim. This thinking has its continuity in the form of seeking treatment from indigenous faith healer like *sadhu, fakir* or *siyane* before coming to the hospital. These healers' practice of treatment is non-scientific. The modes of treatment by these healers include worshipping of gods and deities, and even certain inhuman activities prescribed by them. They also give some *tabeez,* do *jhar-phook* and *tona-totka*. This is all done because women's mental illness is stigmatized more in comparison to men. On the basis of some qualitative information generated from women's case histories, it is found that social and cultural manifestations are so strong that these result in the predisposition of the mental illness among women. They are reflected in form of life events like family breakdown, domestic violence, social pressure and poverty. Exactly 50 per cent of women are dependent exclusively on their husbands. It means it is the husband who is going to decide about the place of the treatment in the patriarchal family system. The access to treatment reveals that nearly 55 per cent of mentally-ill women have come to the hospital of their own, which means they are not referred by any private psychiatrist, or state's post-graduate medical college or any other indigenous faith healer. The mentally-ill women do not have any substance abuse history as only 8 per cent of them are found to be substance abused. It is also interesting to note that 85 per cent of women do not have any history of mental illness. The diagnosis of the mentally-ill patients points out that majority of them are suffering from depression and epilepsy. A substantial number of women are suffering from mental illness for three or more years. It means their treatment is ignored at various levels.

## References

Addlakha, Renu (2001), 'Lay and Medical Diagnoses of Psychiatric Disorder and the Normative Construction of Femininity', in Bhargavi V. Davar (ed.), *Mental Health from a Gender Perspective*, Delhi: Sage Publications.

Chakraborty, Ajitia (1990), *Social Stress and Mental Health: A Social-Psychiatric Field Study of Calcutta*, New Delhi: Sage Publications.

Chandra, Prabha et al. (2003), 'A Cry from the Darkness: Women with Severe Mental Illness in India Reveal their Experiences with Sexual Coercion', *Psychiatry*, Vol. 66, No. 4, pp. 323–34.

Channa, S.M. (1997), 'Gender and Social Space in Haryana Village', *Indian Journal of Gender Studies*, Vol. 4, No. 1, pp. 21–34.

Clark, Russell D. (1989), 'Gender Differences in Receptivity to Sexual Offers', *Journal of Psychology and Human Sexuality*, Vol. 2, No. 1.

Connell, R.W. (1987), *Gender and Power*, Cambridge: Polity Press.

Crothers, Charles (1996), *Social Structure*, London: Routledge.

Davar, V. Bhargavi (1997), 'Sudhir Kakar's Inner World, From the Cross-roads of Philosophy of Science, Feminism and Culture', Unpublished Manuscript.

——. (2000), *Mental Health of Indian Women: A Feminist Agenda*, New Delhi: Sage Publications.

Davar, V. Bhargavi (ed.) (2001), *Mental Health from a Gender Perspective*, New Delhi: Sage Publications.

Dennerstein, Lorraine et al. (1993), 'Menopausal Symptoms in Australian Women', *Medical Journal of Australia*, Vol. 159, pp. 232–36.

Foucault, Michael (2001), *Madness and Civilization*, London: Routledge and Kegan Paul.

Ganguli, H.C. (2000), 'Epidemiological Findings on Prevalence of Mental Disorders in India', *Indian Journal of Psychiatry*, 42(1), January–March, 14–20.

Issac, M.K. and R.L. Kapur (1980), 'A Cost-Effective Analysis of Three Different Methods of Psychiatric Case Finding in General Population', *British Journal of Psychiatry*, Vol. 137, pp. 540–46.

Khan, M.E. et al. (2000), 'Violence against Women and its Impact on Women's Live: Some Observations from Bangladesh', *Journal of Family Welfare*, Vol. 46, pp. 12–24.

Levy, R.I. (1992), 'A Prologue to Psychiatric Anthropology', in T. Schwartz, G.M. White and C.A. Lutz (eds), *New Directory in Psychological Anthropology*, Cambridge: Cambridge University Press.

Mohan, Brij (1966), 'Religion, Superstition and Mental Illness', *Social Work Forum*, Vol. IV, No. 3, Delhi.

Nagla, Madhu (2003), 'Gender Inequality: Perceptive Threat to Health', *Nucleus*, Vol. III, No. 1, January-June.

Nunley, Michael (1998), 'The Involvement of Families in Indian Psychiatry', *Culture, Medicine and Psychiatry*, Vol. 22, No. 3.

Okuma, Truo and Naoko Shimoyama (1972), 'Course of Endogenous Manic Degressive Psychosis, Precipitating Factors and Premorbid Personality: A Statistical Study', *Psychiatry and Clinical Neurosciences*, Vol. 26, Issue 1, 19–33.

Pan American Health Organisation (1995), *The Health Situation of Women in Latin America*, Washington, D.C.

Patel, V. et al.(1999), 'Women, Poverty and Common Mental Disorders in Four Restructuring Societies', *Social Science Medicine*, Vol. 49, No. 11, pp. 1461–71.

——. (2000), *The State of Goa's Health: A Report*, New Delhi: Voluntary Health Association of India.

——. (2006), 'Why Gender Disadvantage and Reproductive Health Risks Factors for Common Mental Diagnosis in Women: A Community

Survey in India', *Archives of General Psychiatry*, Vol. 63, No. 4, pp. 404–13.

Prasad, J. et al. (2003), 'Symptoms Related to the Reproductive Tract and Mental Health among Women in Rural Southern India', *National Medical Journal of India*, Vol. 16, pp. 303–08.

Reddy, M.V. and C.R. Chandrashekar (1988), 'Prevalence of Mental and Behavioural Disorders in India: A Meta Analysis', *Indian Journal of Psychiatry*, 40: 149–57.

Sandhya (1994), *Widowhood: A Socio-psychiatric Study*, Delhi: Mohit Publications.

Sastry, Nalini (1990), 'Anxiety, Sex-role Orientation and Age: Married Women in Urban India', *The Indian Journal of Social Work*, Vol. LI, No. 4, pp. 659–68.

Scheff, J. (1999), *Being Mentally Ill: A Sociological Theory*, New York: Aldine de Gruyter.

Sethi, B.B. (1982), 'A Need for Marriage Counselling', *Indian Journal of Psychiatry*, Vol. 20, No. 3, pp. 283–88.

Sethi, B.B. and R. Manchanda (1978), 'Family Structure and Psychiatric Disorders', *Indian Journal of Psychiatry*, 20(3), 283–288.

Shah, A. (1982), 'Prevalence of Autism and Related Conditions in Adults in a Mental Handicap Hospital', *PubMed*, 3(3): 303–17.

Sharma, V. et al. (1998), 'Can Married Women Say No to Sex? Repercussion of the Denial of Sexual Act', *Journal of Family Welfare*, Vol. 44, pp. 1–8.

Skultans, V. (1991), 'Women and Affliction in Maharashtra: A Hydraulic Model of Health and Illness', *Culture, Medicine and Psychiatry*, Vol. 15, No. 3.

Sonpar, Shobna and Ravi Kapur (1999), 'Non-Conventional Indicators of Gender Disparities Under Structural Reforms', Paper presented at the Workshop on Gender Discrimination Under Structural Reforms, New Delhi: Institute for Social Studies Trust.

Ulrich, H.E. (1987), 'A Study of Change and Depression among Havik Brahmin Women in South Indian Village', *Culture, Medicine and Psychiatry*, Vol. 11, No. 2, pp. 261–87.

World Health Organization (WHO) (2000), *Women's Mental Health: An Evidence Based Review*, Geneva: Switzerland.

——.(2001), *The World Health Report 2001: Mental Health: New Understanding*, New Hope, Geneva: Switzerland.

——.(2003), *Investing in Mental Health*, http://www.who.int/mentalhealth/media/investing-mnh.pdf.

# 11 Women's Perception of Yoga, Health and Leisure

## Yoga as an Alternative Health Care System

Over the centuries, medical wisdom in India evolved within a framework which linked health to a state of harmony, and disease to a state of imbalance. The focus has been on wellness and remaining well, not in fixing the problem after you fall ill.

Unlike allopathy, ayurveda and homeopathy, yoga is not a system of medicine though it enunciates principles through which one can remain healthy and physically fit. Yoga means joining or yoking the individual soul to the universal soul, the union of personal spirit with God. The Sanskrit word *yuj,* from which the word 'yoga' seems to have been derived, means 'to join' or 'to yoke'. The Rigveda hymn tells of an ascetic who achieved supernatural powers by following the yogic path (Radhakrishnan, 1958). The term 'yoga' in its technical sense first occurs in the Taittiriya Upanishad (*Taittiriya Upanishad*, II, Yoga Atma) and the Katha Upanishad (*Katha Upanishad,* II, Adhyatama Yoga). Yogic concepts and techniques remain scattered in the Vedic and Upanishadic literature till about 300 BC. Patanjali collected the old writings and compiled them into his *Yoga Sutras*. He created neither the yoga techniques nor its philosophy; he merely published and corrected. As regards providing theoretical and metaphysical foundation, he made use of the already existing Samkhya philosophy and adapted it to yoga meditation. Woods (1914) opined that in India and in the West the author of the *Yoga Sutras* is also the author of other great works on yoga. This has not been established definitely, but it may be estimated that the relevant works could not have been written later than the 10th century. These works were probably written sometime in the 4th or 5th century AD. Yoga practices are very ancient. Some of the seals recovered at Mohenjo-dara show a divine being sitting in a yogic posture. Rigveda mentions a seer sitting in a yogic asana. Early Upanishad mentions different yogic exercises and procedures. It was Patanjali who around the 3rd century BC systematized all the existing yoga practices. By linking them with the tenets of the Samkhya School of Philosophy, he gave them a regular shape and evolved yoga philosophy. This is enunciated in his *Yoga Sutras*.

The system of yoga enunciated by Patanjali consists of eight components: *yama, niyama, asana, pranayama, pratyahara, dharana, dhyana* and *samadhi*. The first five components relate to the body: they prepare the body for the next three components which relate to mind. The basic tenets are: restrained social behaviour *(yama)*, good personal conduct *(niyama)*, yogic exercises *(asana)*, breathing exercises (*pranayama*), meditation (*dhyana*) and attainment of super-consciousness *(samadhi)*. One can practise them to enable one to achieve sincere selfless service and calmness of mind. These practices are also believed to help in acquiring maximum creative intelligence (Udupa, 1983).

Practice of yoga is neither a Hindu religious dogma nor the monopoly of Indians alone. The pre-requisites of yoga practice are *yama* and *niyama*, not the concepts of any particular religion. Yoga practices are widespread in India and in China, and are also common among the Muslim Sufis and some Christian sects. However, Indian yoga is the most systematic (Udupa, 1983). *Hatha-Yog-Pradinika* texts state that in treating all diseases, the skilful physician should carefully administer treatment according to the methods prescribed by the science of medicine and also administer yogic treatment (Jaggi, 1973).

Yoga is therefore a system of philosophy and health science which has shown positive results in treating certain conditions of stress and psychosomatic illnesses. In this system, no chemical, physical or botanical agent is administered internally. Yoga is regarded as a system of health care which cures mental and physical illness without a great investment of time. While a majority of Indians are familiar with yoga, many think it is too complex and time consuming to practise. The Swami (Ramdev), has become widely popular with a 'yoga made easy' approach that promised to yield quick health benefits with minimal effort (*Dainik Jagran*, 5 September 2005).

## Health Care

People are often awed by modern medicine. The gleaming hospitals, expensive equipment and sophisticated machines are all very impressive and reassuring when you are sick. However, paradoxically, even though medicine has made dramatic advances, many patients are still dissatisfied with medical care today. This has resulted in a move toward 'alternative' medicine, which has become increasingly popular all over the world. In India, which is a bastion of hi-tech scientific medicine, more than 50 per cent of patients have visited an alternative medicine practitioner because they have been unhappy with the care provided by modern medicine (Nagla, 1997). There are many reasons for this state of affairs. Mainstream medicine has become highly commercial, doctors are often too busy to spend time with patients, so the patients say that modern medicine is too impersonal. While it is true that patients need technology, they also, it seems, want tender loving care. Moreover, while modern medicine excels in certain areas (like complex surgery for birth defects and antibiotics for serious infections), it has failed miserably in many areas of disease prevention.

Alternative medicine practitioners, on the other hand, can be very good at this. Often this is all they have to offer, but they offer it very well indeed. They sit down and talk to the patient, touch and feel, ask questions, and all this gives a good feel to the patient. There is no doubt about the efficacy of the placebo effect (Nagla, 1997). Modern medicine treats illnesses using science and technology – it focuses on solving the problem when the patient is sick. Alternative medicine, in a radically different approach, emphasizes the need for patients to take more responsibility for their own health. It is more of an interactive approach. The present chapter focuses on one of the alternative therapies – yoga – a holistic system which links health with the way of life.

Human society has tried to adapt itself for survival through trial and error methods with different types of knowledge in different parts of the world, the offshoots of which include the development of culture, education, scientific knowledge, information systems and the material development of some societies. The chapter deals with yoga as an alternative health care method and how it has created space for women to enhance their health and leisure.

## Women and Leisure

Leisure is a basic need of human life. It provides physical and mental relaxation to person. It is equally important for both man and woman. But, in the Indian society, which is male-dominated, there is a big difference between leisure of men and women. Traditionally, women have always been treated as subordinated to men in every aspect of life. Their place of work is confined to do household chores. They move only within the narrow sphere of kitchen, cooking, child bearing and rearing, and catering to the relatives, in-laws and husband. They have practically no idea of the world outside. On the other hand, the man is attached with the outside world. He is the one who is related with the economic activities of the family by doing job. It is considered that a man has a right of spare time for physical and mental health while woman has no need for it. Various norms and values of society have also limited the leisure activities of women whereas it is not in the case so far as men are concerned.

Leisure researchers have often acted as a prophet of good fortune or doom. Some have predicted a new age of leisure, a society of wealth, and a drastic reduction in working time. Kenneth Roberts (1981) distinguishes an 'optimistic' scenario (increase in wealth, more gratification at work, extended leisure) from a 'pessimistic' scenario (limited growth, ecological constraints). He opts for a moderate scenario: an irrefutable growth in leisure as it occupies a larger space than before. But he reminds us of the danger of generalization. We are not moving towards a society of leisure but towards a society in which leisure is an undeniable and larger component.

Leisure activities for women have changed immeasurably in the last fifty years or so. While men's and children's activities largely involve play and competition, women have seemed to spend whatever leisure time they have had in the productive arts. A grandmother used to say that idle hands were the devil's workshop. Girls were encouraged to knit, sew, embroider or weave. While these activities were necessary for our female ancestors, they took away leisure time as an arena of choice, if indeed any leisure time remained after families had been fed, children bathed and put to bed, and the pile of ironing and mending whittled down. Today, women may choose quilting and other crafts as their favourite leisure time activities. But equally, they can go shopping, to the cinema or participate in kitty parties. And, they can also choose gardening as much for the love of digging into the rich earth as for the pleasure of cooking new varieties of meals.

The evolution of work activities into leisure time hobbies will keep social anthropologists filling books for years to come. So will the social revolutions that lead to profound changes in the very definition of what constitutes leisure time. If mom cooks something extra as a special dish after work, most families recognize that as dinner. If dad spends half of Sunday cooking special lunch fried rice and curry *chhole* (chick peas), we are more likely to identify this as his gourmet-cooking hobby. But, the reverse can also be true if mom has taken up chainsaw sculpture and dad is happily knitting a sweater.

Women's lifestyles and leisure choices are no longer predictable, nor are they static. The passion and interests that are put on hold while women pursue careers, education and family responsibilities may suddenly take root when the nest is empty and time is available. Many women have chosen to include yoga and fitness routines among their lifestyle choices, recognizing the physical and mental health benefits of exercise. The value of recreation and social participation is generally acknowledged, but for no group are these of greater health value than for women.

## Yoga as a Leisure Activity

Human beings have suffered from physical and mental diseases from time immemorial. They have been treated through various types of medicines to cure their physical and mental illnesses. Yoga is a great natural medicine to cure physical and mental pathologies. Yoga medicine is a cost-free leisure activity. It is a self-treatment method which demands understanding and orderliness. It is a process of searching for oneself, self-transcendence and cosmic consciousness. Vedas say that through yoga one is united with God. Likewise, Upanishads tell, 'Yoga is not for weaklings'. According to Patanjali, yoga is the cessation of mind. The aim of yoga is to achieve *kaivalays* or perfect liberation. It is a state of happiness, peace, tranquillity and bliss.

The patient in modern medicine has to do very little or nothing at all. The task of correcting disease and disorder and restoring health is assigned to medicine. There is a contrast here between the modern medical system and the yogic system of treatment. Whereas in the modern medical system it is an external agent (medicine) that does the corrective work, in the yogic system it is the patient himself/herself whose personal understanding, practice and care cure the disease.

In certain cases modern medicine provides immediate relief but not a lasting cure. On the other hand, a great number of patients achieve permanent cures through therapeutic yoga within a period of two to four months. This has been so in cases of diabetes, arthritis, asthma, gastro-intestinal disorders and nervous tension.

Yoga does not involve any expense. It creates a healthy and good life. A healthy life is a good life. Good life is real life. Jiddu Krishnamurti says, 'Real life is doing something which you love to do with your whole being so that there is no inner contradiction, no war between what you are doing and what you think you should do. Life is then a completely integrated process in which there is tremendous joy. But that can happen only when you are not psychologically depending on anybody, or any society, where there is complete detachment inwardly, for only there is the possibility of loving what you do.'

Below we present the results of a survey into how involvement in learning yoga as a leisure activity contributes to the health of a growing number of women.

## Theoretical Paradigm

Leisure is a way of life reflecting more clearly our basic needs and higher potential as human being. More meaningful leisure activities and a wider acceptance of a right to recreation could reduce the significance to us of work and of affluence for its own sake (Hookway, 1978).

Miller and Robinson (1963) believe that leisure and recreation are cultural universals, being found as common elements in the behaviour of individuals in all societies; however Kaplan's (1960) approach explains the functions of leisure. Nakhooda (1961) puts leisure and recreation in the category which involves freedom of choice and voluntary participation in any activity; leisure can be harmful if the right kind of activity is not chosen. In her opinion, to make a judicious use of leisure recreation becomes necessary. In the opinion of Finlay (cited in Butler, 1967) recreation includes many activities that are usually not thought of as play music, drama, the crafts, every free activity and especially creative activity for the enrichment of life. Roberts (1970) states that since in industrial revolution a general process of structural differentiation within society has taken place with special institutions emerging to fulfil the needs such as education and social welfare which were previously catered multipurpose groups and organizations. Leisure is just one amongst man's activities which have been subjected to the process of structural differentiation.

Leisure as a social phenomenon can be understood and explained only in the context of a social organization. Social structure influences the nature and form of leisure and its activities. In a given society, at a particular time, it allows, dictates, or is conducive to, a particular mode of leisure. It not only determines the form and nature of leisure but also the extent and limit of participation; whether any person would be allowed to participate or not would depend on the social status, gender in a given society (Modi, 1985). On the other hand, leisure itself helps in generating new structures and social norms. History abounds in instances which support the contention that social structure influences the nature and form of social norms and generated by leisure.

## Methods

Moving from the question of what is leisure to who is leisure raises real problems for leisure research. What if individual is a woman and not a man? How yoga is her means of deliverance from fatigue and boredom? How far is a woman's choice of yoga turn out to be health and leisure benefiting activity? And, how the decision-making process of attending the yoga camp has liberated her from her household chores for sometime.

The main purpose of the present study is to understand the involvement of women in learning yoga as a leisure activity which in turn contributes to their good health. For this study, we selected Rohtak town in Haryana as the camp was organized there. Rohtak also has an advantage of its proximity with New Delhi, the national capital, which helps in the inflow of information and activities. In all Haryana occupies a status of very well-developed state in India with the second highest per capita income. But, at the same time, in terms of its social index, it is very conservative in the sense that the status of women is very low (Chaudhary, 1993).

The data in this study are based on interviews with women who attended a seven-day yoga activity camp in Rohtak city. The camp was attended by 30,000 people from all parts of the state, along with neighbouring states. Nearly half of them were women. Near the site of the camp is the residential locality, Dev Colony, where nearly every household had at least one guest who came for attending the camp. Therefore, we decided to approach women residents of Dev Colony and their women guests for the interviews. We were thus able to interview 150 women respondents, and gathered information about their socio-economic backgrounds, health-related behaviour, decision-making behaviour for attending yoga camp, and their experiences at the camp. Some questions (regarding socio-economic background, for example) were closed, meaning that there were fixed categories of answers. Other questions were open-ended and yielded more of qualitative information. All the interviews were tape recorded.

The camp was organized by one of the state's leading industrialists in the grounds of Jat College. These grounds have a capacity to accommodate about 50,000 people. The camp was led by the very famous yogic practitioner, Baba Ram Dev Ji, who had been organizing such camps all over India and also had a regular TV broadcast. By local demand, the camps were organized in particular cities with the location and other facilities for accommodating large numbers of people. One such camp was organized in Rohtak city from 25 May to 1 June 2005. Even though Rohtak is very close to Delhi, where the premier medical institutions and hospitals exist. In Rohtak itself there is a big post-graduate medical college and hospital along with a civil hospital. There are numerous private practitioners along with diagnostic facilities. This particular camp was attended by people from different parts of Haryana as well as from neighbouring states like Rajasthan, Punjab, Himachal Pradesh and Delhi. The fees for attending the seven-day yoga camp ranged from ₹ 500 to ₹ 1,500, but there were two days available for people who wanted to attend the camp without paying any fee, and on these days the attendance increased to 50,000. The timing of the yoga camp was from 4 am to 6 am each morning.

## Status of Women

In traditional societies, the status of both individuals and households, as well as access to key social resources, are to a large extent structured by family, marriage and kin relationships. These relationships vary greatly – in fact, the kinship systems of Hindu northern India, Hindu southern India and Muslim India are all different. What is common to them is that they define gender in social terms, that is, the roles, functions and behaviour of men and women within the larger social system.

Two related sets of criteria can be used to assess the status of women within these systems (Basu, 1989; Dyson and Moore, 1983). First, exposure to and interaction with the outside world, which is instrumental in determining the possibilities available to women in their daily lives. Second, the status of women is affected by their degrees of autonomy and capacity to make decisions both inside and outside their households. Autonomy includes the ability to control one's own physical movements, and to acquire, retain, and dispose of earnings, property, etc.

By these criteria, the position of women in northern areas, which also include Haryana, is notably poor (Chaudhary, 1993). Traditional Hindu society in northern rural areas is hierarchical and dominated by men, and its patrilineal, patrilocal structures have implications for women. Restrictions on women's personal movements and interactions with men often amount to *purdah* (literal seclusion or veiling the head and face from public observation). Because emotional ties between spouses are considered a potential threat to the solidarity of the patrilineal group, the northern systems tend to segregate the sexes and limit communication between spouses – a circumstance that has myriad direct and indirect consequences for women's health.

### Social Profile of the Women Who Attended the Yoga Camp

It is clear from Table 1 that most of the women were in the age group ranging from 20 to 60. Actually, they were mostly in the middle age group, which means that they were able to have access to health-promoting activities before reaching old age. Being in this age group they are also partially exempted from taking and thus take care of themselves. Their large attendance could also have been due to the fact that the mid-life group is the most vulnerable from the health point of view as women are still expected to perform all the household chores. The total literacy rate in Haryana is 68.59 per cent but among females it is only 56.31 per cent which is below the national average (Census of India, 2001). Our study shows that the women who attended the camp were mostly literate. Only 13 (8.66%) were illiterate. It is interesting to note that, among the literates, 57 (38%) had professional education while another 42 (28%) were graduates or post-graduates, whereas only 38 (25.33%) were between primary and higher secondary. It was also found that the majority of the respondents, i.e., 129 (86%), belonged to the nuclear family as against 21 (14%) who came from joint family background. The table also reveals that just 11 (7.33%) had income below ₹ 5,000, 36 (24%) had family income ranging between ₹ 5,001 and ₹ 10,000, and 55 (36.66%) had monthly income in excess of ₹ 20,000. There were only 8 (5.33%) women who occupied administrative, executive or managerial positions, whereas 25 (16.66%) were housewives. The largest group of the women (64, 42.66%) was engaged in clerical and allied work, and 53 (36.33%) were either teacher or doctor. Their working hours also varied but on average they were spending about 6–7 hours per day attending to household chores which included washing clothes, preparing meals, fetching water from handpumps or wells, and in some cases milking buffaloes.

**Table 1** ***Socio-economic profile of the women respondents***

| *Age group* | *20–30 yrs*<br>*28 (18.66)* | *31–40 yrs*<br>*35 (23.33)* | *41–50 yrs*<br>*64 (42.66)* | *51–60 yrs*<br>*23 (15.33)* | *Total*<br>*150 (100)* |
|---|---|---|---|---|---|
| Marital status | Married<br>125 (83.33) | Unmarried<br>17 (11.33) | Widow<br>8 (5.33) | | 150 (100) |
| Education | Illiterate<br>13 (8.66) | Primary<br>Higher Secondary<br>38 (25.33) | Graduation<br>Post-graduation<br>42 (28) | Professional<br>57 (38) | 150 (100) |
| Family | Nuclear<br>129 (86) | Joint<br>21 (14) | | | 150 (100) |
| Monthly income | Below ₹ 5,000<br>11 (7.33) | ₹ 5,001–10,000<br>36 (24) | Rs. 10,001–20,000<br>48 (32) | More than ₹ 20,000<br>55 (36.66) | 150 (100) |
| Occupation | Housewife<br>25 (16.66) | Clerical and allied work<br>64 (42.66) | Professionals<br>(teachers, doctors, etc.)<br>53 (36.33) | Administrative, executive,<br>managerial positions<br>8 (5.33) | 150 (100) |

Figures in parentheses are percentages.

## Listening to and Talking with Women about Health

Reviewing human history in India, it has been observed that women die young, in childbirth or in ill health. They are often victims of abuse, torture, violence, neglect and other forms of social discrimination. Even in today's modern scientific world, the same situation prevails due to the dominance of a complex socio-cultural web which has conditioned women not to complain but to cope silently with their multifaceted health problems (Rajeshwari, 1996).

A bird's eye view of the perilous path that a woman undergoes through her life indicates that as a child she is usually discriminated against and/or overprotected. Robbed of her golden years as young woman, in the anxiety of early marriage, she bears the burden of becoming a mother even before she completes adolescence. The adult personality of an Indian woman is moulded by the society's manipulation of cultural norms, and leads to chronic feelings of low self-esteem. Women are rarely equipped with the courage and confidence to voice any of their problems, including those related to health. By clinging to the hope that their health problems will disappear one day, women lose their adulthood and enter into premature old age without understanding that by then it is too late for treatment.

Discrimination throughout adolescence conditions adult women to fit into the rigidly stereotyped socio-cultural and economic roles laid out for them. They suffer from various general and reproductive health problems. Various socio-economic factors, such as fears of health check-ups, which are not sensitively done and involve strangers, prevent women from seeking timely treatment. The yoga camp had provided them with an opportunity to benefit by coming out from their homes for a week for their own mental and physical well-being.

## Yoga and Outdoor Activities

It is not always possible to establish a distinction between the so-called sports-related and other physical outdoor activities. The available data allows us to conclude that, at least in the West, the practice of traditional sports has stayed relatively steady over time or has even decreased. On the other hand, new activities related to, for instance, physical exercise or the outdoor activities, have risen in popularity. Most popular are usually walking for exercise, swimming and home exercise (Pronovost, 1998). Havighurst (1957) recorded the difference in leisure usage by classes of people – age, sex, economic status and the like. He found that in the middle age women were inclined to concentrate on reading while men were more interested in gardening. A large proportion of the population in the West now regularly do exercises. Most surveys indicate that in the last few decades there has been a growth as well as diversification of sports-related activities that have been integrated into people's lifestyles. In certain segments of the population, it has become part of the daily routine, imposing itself as a behavioural norm, while in others it has become a regular activity, seen as a form of relaxation, entertainment or escape.

The pursuit of a number of outdoor leisure activities may be either for the sake of the context or some specific practice. But, in almost all cases, the attribute 'outdoor' combines with other features so that they become socio-cultural or sports- or family-related activities. It is undeniable that there has been a quantitative growth in outdoor leisure in the last few decades. This is in response to a growing infatuation with the practice of outdoor activities. Rates of participation have undeniably increased significantly. This phenomenon shows a deep transformation in lifestyles and a stronger sensitivity to the natural environment. The pursuit of information and education is an integral part of coming into contact with one's natural surroundings. In the present study also, the men and women alike had decided to attend the yoga camp not only from the leisure activity point of view but also from environmental and health points of view.

## Decision-making

Work and leisure do comprise different sets of activities but these activities are closely related. In the case of work, activities are goal-oriented and the demands placed on individuals are normally demands from an outside agency. In the case of leisure, the activities are decided by the individual himself/herself. Any control there is upon the individual can be manipulated by him/her in the leisure situation. This implies that there is freedom in leisure but that is not present in work (Dunkerley, 1975). Conversely, Roberts (1983) stresses and explains the persistence of class and gender divisions through trends in clothing, music and hair artistry and predicts that these patterns will survive current change. He also explains how leisure education and provision can modify broader patterns and enable all young people to explain the leisure opportunities that their circumstances allow.

If we look at the decision-making behaviour for attending the yoga camp, it is evident from Table 2 that 58 respondents (38.66%) reported that their husbands decided for them, and another 19 (12.66%) mentioned that the head of the household (either father-in-law or elder brother-in-law) had decided for them. It has also been found by Nagla (2003) that, in Haryana, husbands play a dominant role in all categories of household decisions. However, women's employment helps them gain some control over financial matters and decisions related to other household activities. This study also reveals that 46 women (30.66%) had jointly (husband and wife) decided to attend the yoga camp. But, they had to make efforts to persuade their husbands. Although they felt that both men and women were equal, this was only notional in their actual lives. It was always husband who dominated the scene. This is despite the rapid transformation in India that has helped women to assert and take their own decisions concerning themselves and their families. The data reveal that just 21 (14%) of the women had taken the decision by themselves to attend the yoga camp, and of these 5 (3.5%) were widows. When children become adults, they also participate in household decision-making as 6 (4%) of the respondents had been prompted by children to attend yoga camp for health and leisure reasons.

**Table 2** ***Decision-making for attending the yoga camp***

| *Decision taken to attending the yoga camp by* | *Number of respondents* | *Percentage* |
|---|---|---|
| Head of the household, i.e., male member | 19 | 12.66 |
| Husband | 58 | 38.66 |
| Wife | 21 | 14.00 |
| Jointly both husband and wife | 46 | 30.66 |
| Input from adult children | 06 | 4.00 |
| Total | 150 | 100.00 |

## The Gender Division of Yoga Activity

For decades women in India have undertaken household chores, agricultural work like sowing, weeding and cutting as well as lighter physical tasks. We do not have sufficient data to substantiate it, but it seems that the field of 'classical' cultural activities (museums, theatres, concerts) involves more men than women (Pronovost, 1998). This also applies to physical activities. For example, learning and practising yoga have been heavily masculinized. Hochschild (1983) in her study of air hostesses found that human emotional and caring labour, which is assumed to come naturally to women, is commercialized as in the case of air hostess. But, when the uniform or skin is removed, a space is created where there is a need to express both hidden and sincere emotions.

In terms of physical activity, traditionally, women in India grind cereals, fetch water from wells, and collect fuel and fodder from forests and other distant places. They sometimes swim and play games like kho-kho and skipping whereas men prefer wrestling, jumping, all outdoor sports, and yoga too. There is certainly a gender differentiation with regard to participation in yoga activity. The differences are reflected in the Table 3. These differences reflect socialization into traditional family roles.

**Table 3** ***Opinions of women respondents about yoga as feminine/masculine***

| *Characterization of yoga* | *Number of respondents* | *Percentage* |
|---|---|---|
| Feminine | 27 | 18 |
| Masculine | 63 | 42 |
| Gender neutral | 60 | 40 |
| Total | 150 | 100.00 |

We tried to seek the opinions of women respondents regarding yoga as a feminine or masculine activity. The responses were varied. Although the highest number of women, i.e., 63 (42%), opined that yoga was a masculine activity, 27 (18%) differed and argued that it was the only physical leisure time activity which could be performed by women inside the home and so was feminine. Dynamism prevails in India in the opinions of the women respondents (60, 40%) who reported that yoga was gender-neutral.

It has been observed by the Powell and Graves (2003) that parents, teachers and the media play very important roles in shaping children's behaviour. To explore the importance of motivating factors, we asked our respondents who had motivated them to join the yoga camp, and the sources indicated by them are shown in Table 4 below:

**Table 4** ***Sources of information about attending the yoga camp***

| *Source of information* | *Number of respondents* | *Percentage* |
|---|---|---|
| Television | 92 | 61.33 |
| Posters | 23 | 15.33 |
| Newspapers | 25 | 16.66 |
| Family and/or friends | 10 | 6.66 |
| Total | 150 | 100.00 |

As many as 92 (61.33%) of the respondents had obtained information through television, 23 (15.33%) through posters, and 25 (16.66%) through newspapers. Only 10 (6.66%) had gathered information from their families or from friends. Deem and Gilory (1998) stressed that strategies should be formulated to encourage women to engage in physical activity using a wider concept of physical activity, examining its location within broader notion of women's leisure, and exploring how physical activities relates to sexuality and empowerment of individual.

## Reasons for Attending

Sociologically speaking, no action is performed without any objective, although the objective can be manifest or latent. Yoga as an alternative form of health care is rapidly making inroads not only as a physical activity to keep oneself mentally and physically fit but also for bringing people out, particularly women, from their homes onto open ground for learning and practice.

It has been observed that more and more people are opting for yoga. There is a dynamic interaction of diverse factors that influence women in unique ways in their decisions to join yoga camps. Table 5 shows that most of the women mentioned more than one reason for attending the camp. Typically, the respondents (83, 55.33%) had joined the camp because their primary concern was to cure illnesses, but 124 (82.66%) were interested in keeping themselves physically and mentally fit, and free from tensions and worries. It is interesting to note that a sizeable number of women (87 or 58%) just wanted to go outside their homes for relief from monotonous daily life. The yoga camp then opened outlets for them to go daily outside either to parks or elsewhere for practice and to get the chance to meet friends. Otherwise it was very difficult for the women to go outside without any good reason. A few, but still 34 or 22.66 per cent, simply wanted to try something new in their lives by attending the yoga camp.

**Table 5** ***Reasons for attending the camp***

| *Reasons for attending the yoga camp* | *Number of respondents** | *Percentage* |
|---|---|---|
| To get rid of diseases | 83 | 55.33 |
| To keep oneself physically and mentally fit | 124 | 82.66 |
| Wanted to go outside for leisure | 87 | 58.00 |
| To try something new in life | 34 | 22.66 |
| By attending I can go daily to the park | 62 | 41.33 |

* Multiple responses permitted.

## Flexitime

Hard and regular physical activity may bring disenchantment to life. But if it is not taken only as a leisure activity, but also for some health philosophy, then it has to be followed according to some rules and regulations. In this context, we asked our women about flexibility in the timing of their yoga activity. All the women agreed that attending a particular camp had to be at a fixed time. However, after attending the yoga camp, practising on their own could be flexible, as 85 (56.66%) of the women reported that they then did not feel pressure or time constraints. Opposing this, 65 (43.33%) of the women felt strongly that there should be some fixed time for yoga activity otherwise it would lose its importance from the health point of view (Table 6).

**Table 6** ***Flexibility of time in yoga practice***

| *Prefer flexibility of Time* | *Number of respondents* | *Percentage* |
|---|---|---|
| Yes | 85 | 56.66 |
| No | 65 | 43.33 |
| Total | 150 | 100.00 |

## Experience of Attending Yoga

There is a commonsense tendency to use stereotyped expressions to legitimize any behaviour. Yoga is one physical activity which has been legitimized as health care, for keeping oneself physically and mentally fit. One of the most accepted 'facts' in sociology and anthropology is that any society is dependent on the existence of a general 'cultural system' from which individuals, groups and institutions draw their legitimacy. It is claimed that there must be a symbolic system, of whatever kind, a basis for social behaviour. And, at the core of this 'cultural system' there are said to be values. Values are said to play an essential role in society. They form the basis of the actors' interpretations and ultimate judgements on social reality. They indicate ideal ways of thinking and acting. They focus on what is considered desirable and essential within a given society. They lay the foundations of patterns of behaviour, and of the normative orientations of social action. They thereby contribute to societal coherence. The structure of values is, however, specific to a given society, at a given historical moment and within given collectivities. Many leisure scholars and researchers maintain that leisure is the source of the rise of new values and changes in modern societies. Dumazedier (1967) has assembled a number of findings from his study to frame for supporting his contention that the effect of leisure on work is now more marked than vice-versa. Parker (1976) found that influence of leisure on work is witnessed in the sense that there is a substantial growth in leisure industry which includes entertainment, sports and gambling, holiday amenities, care of gardens and pets and so on. Yoga activity is a departure from hurry and worry, therefore, a form of leisure activity. Our study tried to focus on how yoga as a physical activity has also turned out to be a leisure activity. The results are presented below in Table 7:

**Table 7** ***Overall experience of attending the yoga camp***

| *Overall Experience* | *Number of Respondents** | *Percentage* |
|---|---|---|
| Feeling physically healthy | 90 | 60.00 |
| Feeling mentally healthy | 62 | 41.33 |
| Feeling physically and mentally healthy | 117 | 78.00 |
| Social time for self | 43 | 28.66 |
| Experience of pleasure | 51 | 34.00 |
| Individual liberty | 39 | 26.00 |

*Multiple responses permitted.

The answers came in multiple response form. The data reveal that the majority of respondents (117, 78%) it found it a way to keep themselves physically and mentally healthy which further affected their roles in the family. Forty-three or 28.66 per cent said that by attending yoga they could find social time for themselves, and 51 (34%) reported that it provided them an experience of pleasure. Thirty-nine (26%) viewed yoga as a form of individual liberation.

## Conclusion

The study of yoga health activity is important for understanding a number of fundamental dynamics underlying cultural questions. Our study notably reveals the inseparability between the values of society and the changing perceptions of women in asserting health and leisure values. This study helps to document a major new health-related activity, i.e., yoga practice, which challenges conventional gender divisions in leisure and is a source of information on health. It alerts, it individualizes, and allows flexibility in the use of time. This diversification of values makes yoga not only a means of physical and mental therapy but also an important leisure activity, particularly for women, in India.

It may be stated that leisure, yoga and health are essentially associated with the nature of social organization and the leisure activities as established in society by its cultural and structural correlates.

## References

Basu, Alkia (1989), 'Cultural Differences in the Status of Women in India', in A. Bose and P. Desai (eds), *Population Transition in India*, New Delhi: B.R. Publishing Corporation.

Census of India (2001), *Population Tables*, New Delhi: Government of India.

Chaudhary, Prem (1993), 'High Participation, Low Evaluation: Women and Work in Rural Haryana', *Economic and Political Weekly*, Vol. 28, No. 52, 25 December.

Deem, Rosemary and Sarah Gilory (1998), 'Physical Activity, Life-long Learning and Empowerment: Studying Sport in Women's Leisure', *Sport, Education and Society*, Vol. 46, No. 7.

Dumazedier, Joffre (1967), *Towards a Society of Leisure*, London: Collier Macmillan.

Dunkerley, David (1975), *Occupation and Society*, London: Routledge.

Dyson, T. and M. Moore (1983), 'On Kinship Structure, Female Autonomy and Demographic Behaviour in India', *Population and Development Review*, Vol. 9, No. 1, pp. 5–60.

English Homeopathy Association (1847), 'Medical Prejudices', Delhi.

Finlay, John H., cited in George D. Butler (1967), *Introduction to Community Recreation*, New York: McGraw-Hill Book Co., p. 3.

Havighurst, Robert J. (1957), 'The Leisure Activities of the Middle Aged', *American Journal of Sociology*, Vol. LXII, No. 2, September.

Hochschild (1983), 'A Study of Airline Hostesses', *Sociological Abstract*, Vol. 48, No. 3.

Hookway, R. (1978), *Issues in Recreation*, England: Penguin Books Ltd.

Jaggi, O.P. (1973), *Yogic and Tantric Medicine*, Vol. V, Delhi: Atma Ram and Sons.

Kaplan, Max (1960), *Leisure in America: A Social Inquiry*, New York: John Wiley and Sons, Inc.

Miller, Norman and Dunae M. Robinson (1963), *The Leisure Age: Its Challenge to Recreation*, California: Wadsworth Publishing Company, Inc.

Modi, Ishwar (1985), *Leisure, Mass Media and Social Structure*, Jaipur: Rawat Publications.

Nagla, Madhu (1997), *Sociology of Medical Profession: A Study of Medical Organizations and Profession of Medicine in Haryana*, Jaipur: Rawat Publications.

——. (2003), 'Gender Inequality: Perceptive Threat to Health', *Nucleus*, Vol. III, No. 1, January-June.

Nakhooda, Zulie (1961), *Leisure and Recreation in Society*, Allahabad: Kitab Mahal.

Neumeyer, Martin H. and Esther S. Neumeyer (1968), *Leisure and Recreation: A Study of Leisure and Recreation in their Sociological Aspects*, New York: Ronald Press Company.

Parker, S. (1976), *The Sociology of Leisure*, London: Allen and Unwin.

Pronovost, Gilles (1998), 'The Sociology of Leisure', *Current Sociology*, Vol. 46, No. 3, July.

Powell, G.N. and L.M. Graves (2003), *Women and Men in Management*, New Delhi: Sage Publications.

Radhakrishnan, S. (1958), *Indian Philosophy*, London: George Allen & Unwin.

Rajeshwari (1996), 'Gender Bias in Utilization of Health Care Facilities in Rural Haryana', *Economic and Political Weekly*, Vol. 31, No. 8.

Roberts, Kenneth (1970), *Leisure: Aspects of Modern Society*, London: Prentice Hall Press.

——. (1981), *Leisure*, London: Longman.

——. (1983), *Youth and Leisure*, London: George Allen and Unwin.

Sadar (1996), 'Social and Material Determinants of Leisure', *Sociological Abstract*, Vol. 35, No. 6.

Udupa, K.N. (1983), Presidential Address on the Occasion of the Asian Congress of the Indian Association for Traditional Asian Medicine, held at Bombay, 6–9 March.

Woods, J.H. (1914), *The Yoga-System of Patanjali*, Harvard Oriental Series, Delhi: Motilal Banarsidass.

Zuzanek, Jiri and Roger Mannell (1983), 'Work-Leisure Relationship from a Sociological and Social Psychological Perspective', *Leisure Studes*, Vol. 2, No. 3, pp. 327–44.

# Index